Soft Tissue Surgery

Editors

LISA M. HOWE
HARRY W. BOOTHE Jr

VETERINARY CLINICS OF NORTH AMERICA: SMALL ANIMAL PRACTICE

www.vetsmall.theclinics.com

May 2015 • Volume 45 • Number 3

ELSEVIER

1600 John F. Kennedy Boulevard • Suite 1800 • Philadelphia, Pennsylvania, 19103-2899
http://www.vetsmall.theclinics.com

VETERINARY CLINICS OF NORTH AMERICA: SMALL ANIMAL PRACTICE Volume 45, Number 3
May 2015 ISSN 0195-5616, ISBN-13: 978-0-323-37625-9

Editor: Patrick Manley
Developmental Editor: Meredith Clinton

Veterinary Clinics of North America: Small Animal Practice (ISSN 0195-5616) is published bimonthly by Elsevier Inc., 360 Park Avenue South, New York, NY 10010-1710. Months of issue are January, March, May, July, September, and November. Business and Editorial Offices: 1600 John F. Kennedy Blvd., Ste. 1800, Philadelphia, PA 19103-2899. Customer Service Office: 3251 Riverport Lane, Maryland Heights, MO 63043. Periodicals postage paid at New York, NY and additional mailing offices. Subscription prices are $310.00 per year (domestic individuals), $500.00 per year (domestic institutions), $150.00 per year (domestic students/residents), $410.00 per year (Canadian individuals), $621.00 per year (Canadian institutions), $455.00 per year (international individuals), $621.00 per year (international institutions), and $220.00 per year (international and Canadian students/residents). To receive student/resident rate, orders must be accompanied by name of affiliated institution, date of term, and the *signature* of program/residency coordinator on institution letterhead. Orders will be billed at individual rate until proof of status is received. Foreign air speed delivery is included in all *Clinics* subscription prices. All prices are subject to change without notice. **POSTMASTER:** Send address changes to *Veterinary Clinics of North America: Small Animal Practice*, Elsevier Health Sciences Division, Subscription Customer Service, 3251 Riverport Lane, Maryland Heights, MO 63043. Customer Service (orders, claims, online, change of address): Elsevier Periodicals Customer Service, Elsevier Health Sciences Division Subscription Customer Service 3251 Riverport Lane Maryland Heights, MO 63043. Tel: 1-800-654-2452 (U.S. and Canada); 314-447-8871 (outside U.S. and Canada). Fax: 314-447-8029. E-mail: journalscustomerservice-usa@elsevier.com (for print support); journalsonlinesupport-usa@elsevier.com (for online support).

Reprints. For copies of 100 or more of articles in this publication, please contact the Commercial Reprints Department, Elsevier Inc., 360 Park Avenue South, New York, NY 10010-1710. Tel.: 212-633-3874; Fax: 212-633-3820; E-mail: reprints@elsevier.com.

Veterinary Clinics of North America: Small Animal Practice is also published in Japanese by Inter Zoo Publishing Co., Ltd., Aoyama Crystal-Bldg 5F, 3-5-12 Kitaaoyama, Minato-ku, Tokyo 107-0061, Japan.

Veterinary Clinics of North America: Small Animal Practice is covered in *Current Contents/Agriculture, Biology and Environmental Sciences, Science Citation Index, ASCA, MEDLINE/PubMed (Index Medicus), Excerpta Medica, and BIOSIS.*

Contributors

EDITORS

LISA M. HOWE, DVM, PhD
Diplomate, American College of Veterinary Surgeons; Professor of Small Animal Surgery, Department of Small Animal Clinical Sciences, College of Veterinary Medicine and Biomedical Sciences, Texas A&M University, College Station, Texas

HARRY W. BOOTHE Jr, DVM, MS
Diplomate, American College of Veterinary Surgeons; Professor and Surgery Section Chief of Small Animal Surgery, Department of Clinical Sciences, Wilford and Kate Bailey Small Animal Teaching Hospital, College of Veterinary Medicine, Auburn University, Auburn, Alabama

AUTHORS

DAWN MERTON BOOTHE, DVM, PhD
Diplomate, American College of Veterinary Internal Medicine; Diplomate, American College of Veterinary Clinical Pharmacology; Professor and Director, Clinical Pharmacology Laboratory, Department of Anatomy, Physiology and Pharmacology, College of Veterinary Medicine, Auburn University, Auburn, Alabama

HARRY W. BOOTHE Jr, DVM, MS
Diplomate, American College of Veterinary Surgeons; Professor and Surgery Section Chief of Small Animal Surgery, Department of Clinical Sciences, Wilford and Kate Bailey Small Animal Teaching Hospital, College of Veterinary Medicine, Auburn University, Auburn, Alabama

JACQUELINE R. DAVIDSON, DVM, MS
Diplomate, American College of Veterinary Surgeons; Diplomate, American College of Veterinary Sports Medicine and Rehabilitation; Clinical Professor, College of Veterinary Medicine and Biomedical Sciences, Texas A&M University, College Station, Texas

LISA M. HOWE, DVM, PhD
Diplomate, American College of Veterinary Surgeons; Professor of Small Animal Surgery, Department of Small Animal Clinical Sciences, College of Veterinary Medicine and Biomedical Sciences, Texas A&M University, College Station, Texas

BRAD M. MATZ, DVM, MS
Diplomate, American College of Veterinary Surgeons - Small Animal; ACVS Fellow, Assistant Clinical Professor, Surgical Oncology, Department of Clinical Sciences, Auburn University, Auburn, Alabama

MILAN MILOVANCEV, DVM
Diplomate, American College of Veterinary Surgeons - Small Animal; Assistant Professor, Small Animal Surgery; Department of Clinical Sciences, College of Veterinary Medicine, Oregon State University, Corvallis, Oregon

LAURA E. PEYCKE, DVM, MS
Diplomate, American College of Veterinary Surgeons; Diplomate, American College of Sport Medicine and Rehabilitation; Clinical Associate Professor, Department of Veterinary Small Animal Clinical Sciences, College of Veterinary Medicine and Biomedical Sciences, Texas A&M University, College Station, Texas

MARYANN RADLINSKY, DVM, MS
Diplomate, American College of Veterinary Surgeons; Associate Professor, Small Animal Medicine and Surgery, College of Veterinary Medicine, The University of Georgia, Athens, Georgia

KELLEY M. THIEMAN MANKIN, DVM, MS
Diplomate, American College of Veterinary Surgeons - Small Animal; Assistant Professor, Department of Small Animal Clinical Sciences, College of Veterinary Medicine and Biomedical Sciences, Texas A&M University, College Station, Texas

DAVID MICHAEL TILLSON, DVM, MS
Diplomate, American College of Veterinary Surgeons; Professor, Department of Clinical Sciences, Bailey Small Animal Teaching Hospital, Arthur and Louise Oriole Professor, College of Veterinary Medicine, Auburn University, Auburn, Alabama

KATY L. TOWNSEND, BVSc, MS
Diplomate, American College of Veterinary Surgeons - Small Animal; Department of Clinical Sciences, College of Veterinary Medicine, Oregon State University, Corvallis, Oregon

Contents

can be found in different locations in both small and large breed dogs. Most CPSS are best managed surgically. The goal of surgical management of CPSS is to slowly redirect blood from the shunting vessel through the portal vasculature while avoiding portal hypertension. Many surgical management methods are available, including open and less invasive procedures, such as laparoscopy and embolization.

Thoracic surgery is a challenge for any veterinary surgeon. A review of several important articles on topics relative to thoracotomy procedures is presented. Discussion also includes an evaluation of availability of appropriate surgical facilities, necessary equipment before undertaking thoracic surgical procedures, and the essentials and pitfalls to making an approach and effectively closing the thoracic cavity of a dog or cat. This article reviews the 3 primary types of thoracotomy: lateral (intercostal) thoracotomy, median sternotomy, and transdiaphragmatic thoracotomy. Essential anatomy, surgical approach, and various techniques to ensure effective and durable thoracotomy closure are presented.

Minimally invasive surgery of the abdomen constitutes an increasingly common and developed set of surgical options in small animal veterinary patients. In addition to established procedures, such as laparoscopic gonadectomy and biopsies, more advanced procedures, such as adrenalectomy, cholecystectomy, cisterna chyli ablation, and lymph node extirpation, are described. Some laparoscopic procedures have been reported using different techniques or approaches, reflecting the field's progression beyond its infancy. Advances in equipment and experience among an ever-growing group of veterinary surgeons are expected to result in progressively more widespread adoption of minimally invasive procedures.

Thoracoscopy is a technique that has been shown to decrease patient morbidity and is rapidly becoming more diversely applied for diagnostic and therapeutic interventions in veterinary medicine. This article describes the basic equipment and application of thoracoscopy in small animal surgery. The diagnostic and therapeutic applications are introduced and briefly described.

Current concepts in wound management are summarized. The emphasis is on selection of the contact layer of the bandage to promote a moist wound environment. Selection of an appropriate contact layer is based on the stage of wound healing and the amount of wound exudate. The contact layer can be used to promote autolytic debridement and enhance wound healing.

Lisa M. Howe

Negative pressure wound therapy (NPWT) is becoming recognized in veterinary medicine as a viable option for the management of complex wounds. NPWT has many advantages over traditional wound care and results in quicker and improved wound healing in many instances. This article discusses the art and science of NPWT, as well as the many current indications, complications, advantages and disadvantages, and future directions of NPWT in small animal veterinary medicine. This therapy will likely have a growing role in veterinary medical practice for complicated wound management and other usages in coming years.

Dawn Merton Boothe and Harry W. Boothe Jr

Surgical site infections are among the complications that can be reduced with the timely implementation of appropriate antimicrobial therapy. A 3-D approach to judicious antimicrobial use focuses on the de-escalation of systemic antimicrobial therapy, design of dosing regimens, and decontamination of the surgeon, patient, and environment. De-escalation can be accomplished in part through proper antimicrobial prophylaxis. Dosing regimens should be designed to maximize efficacy and minimize resistance. Decontamination includes disinfection of inanimate surfaces and timely application of appropriate antiseptics at concentrations that maximize efficacy.

VETERINARY CLINICS OF NORTH AMERICA: SMALL ANIMAL PRACTICE

THE CLINICS ARE NOW AVAILABLE ONLINE!
Access your subscription at:
www.theclinics.com

Preface

Soft Tissue Surgery: A Rapidly Evolving Field

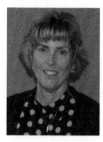 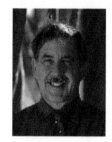

Lisa M. Howe, DVM, PhD, DACVS   Harry W. Boothe Jr, DVM, MS, DACVS
Editors

The field of small animal surgery has undergone a rapid evolution that has seen numerous techniques and practices being developed in and introduced to companion animal surgery. Such evolution often has been brought about because of adaptation of practices used in human surgery for use in companion animals. In addition, many of today's clients have come to expect a level of sophistication in small animal surgery that rivals that of human surgery.

This issue focuses on current concepts of soft tissue surgery and associated subjects. The first article discusses current concepts in oncologic surgery, followed by a discussion of surgical staplers and vessel sealing devices that facilitate oncologic surgery as well as a host of other soft tissue procedures. This is followed by articles examining current concepts in hepatobiliary surgery (an unforgiving and often surgically challenging organ system) and portosystemic shunt surgery, for which the perfect surgical solution has yet to be identified. Surgery of the thorax is then discussed focusing on the practical steps and concepts that are important to consider when performing thoracic surgery. Next, current concepts in minimally invasive surgery of the abdomen and thorax are examined. Understanding of the principles of and indications for minimally invasive surgery is becoming increasingly important as more practices are incorporating minimally invasive surgery as part of their repertoire for soft tissue surgery. Wounds and their management remain a daily part of small animal practice and are discussed in two articles, one that discusses wound management and newer wound-healing products and the other article that examines equipment and techniques of negative pressure wound therapy. Finally, the soft tissue surgeon is more frequently encountering multidrug-resistant organisms and infections, and responsible perioperative antimicrobial usage is critically important in veterinary medicine, as it has been with human medicine. This topic is discussed in the final article.

Vet Clin Small Anim 45 (2015) ix–x
http://dx.doi.org/10.1016/j.cvsm.2015.02.011
0195-5616/15/$ – see front matter © 2015 Published by Elsevier Inc.
vetsmall.theclinics.com

It is our hope that the topics chosen are timely and that this issue will be useful for both the practitioner and specialist who performs small animal soft tissue surgery. We thank our surgical and clinical pharmacologic colleagues for their excellent contributions to this issue.

Lisa M. Howe, DVM, PhD, DACVS
Department of Veterinary Small Animal Clinical Sciences
College of Veterinary Medicine and Biomedical Sciences
Texas A&M University
College Station, TX 77843-4474, USA

Harry W. Boothe Jr, DVM, MS, DACVS
Department of Clinical Sciences
College of Veterinary Medicine
Auburn University
1220 Wire Road
Auburn, AL 36849-5540, USA

E-mail addresses:
lhowe@cvm.tamu.edu (L.M. Howe)
boothhw@auburn.edu (H.W. Boothe)

Current Concepts in Oncologic Surgery in Small Animals

Brad M. Matz, DVM, MS

KEYWORDS

- Mast cell tumors • Soft tissue sarcomas • Injection site sarcomas • Surgical margins
- Surgical oncology • Metronomic chemotherapy

KEY POINTS

- Normal-appearing liver and spleen on ultrasound should still be aspirated.
- A sentinel lymph node is the first lymph node to receive drainage from a tumor; it can reliably be determined with scintigraphy.
- Best recommendations for mast cell tumors (MCTs) margins are difficult to determine. A proportional margin allows surgeons to tailor the margin to patients, and previously recommended margins may be larger than necessary.
- Recently described surgical margins for feline injection site sarcomas are 5 cm lateral and 2 fascial planes deep to the tumor.

MAST CELL TUMORS

Introduction

MCTs are a common clinical diagnosis and are one of the most often encountered cutaneous neoplasms of dogs, ranging from 7% to 21%.[1–4] Several important advancements regarding the staging, treatment, and histologic grading of MCTs have been made and are summarized. Staging is valuable to clinicians because this information has an impact on the pre- and postoperative management of patients. Staging results may also have an impact on the surgical procedure performed on an animal and help prepare the owner for adjuvant therapy that may follow the surgical treatment.

Staging

Introduction

Procedures recommended and organs evaluated in the staging of MCTs are somewhat inconsistent but typically involve sampling the liver, spleen, bone marrow and draining the lymph node, if not other lymph nodes.[5] Staging decisions are

The author has nothing to disclose.
Surgical Oncology, Department of Clinical Sciences, Auburn University, 1220 Wire Road, Auburn, AL 36849-5540, USA
E-mail address: bmm0007@tigermail.auburn.edu

Vet Clin Small Anim 45 (2015) 437–449
http://dx.doi.org/10.1016/j.cvsm.2015.01.003   **vetsmall.theclinics.com**

frequently based on tumor grade because grade 1 MCTs are unlikely to metastasize and dogs are not likely to need full staging, whereas grade 3 MCTs are likely to metastasize and dogs would benefit from staging. The behavior of grade 2 MCT's can be difficult to predict. Histologic features that have been associated with more aggressive behavior are mitotic index, tumor size, and lymph node status.[6]

Technique

Ultrasonographic appearance of the liver and spleen should be interpreted with caution. A study evaluating the correlation of ultrasound findings to cytology evaluated 19 dogs[5]; 10 had grade 2 disease and 9 had grade 3 disease. Sonographic appearance of the spleen and liver was judged normal in 56% and 89%, respectively. All splenic and 14 of 19 liver samples were of diagnostic quality. Splenic and liver involvement was detected in 37% and 16%, respectively. All dogs (3/3) with liver involvement had splenic involvement. Ultrasonographic abnormalities were found in 43% of spleens evaluated and no livers in dogs with cytologic evidence of MCT. Another study similarly recommended aspiration of the liver and spleen despite their appearance. These findings highlight the importance of fine-needle aspiration and not relying on appearance alone.[7]

Bone Marrow

Bone marrow involvement with MCTs generally results in a poor clinical outcome. A study evaluated 14 dogs with bone marrow involvement and found a median survival time (MST) of 43 days.[8] Dogs with bone marrow involvement in this study did not benefit from treatment with lomustine.

Lymph Node Status

Introduction

As stated previously, evaluation of the local lymph node is an important part of clinical staging for determining status of the disease and has a significant impact on prognosis and patient survival. A complete discussion of lymphology is beyond the context of this article but some basic understanding of lymphatic drainage and lymphocentrums is important to the understanding of lymph node staging. A lymphocentrum is a lymph node or group of lymph nodes in the same region that receives afferent lymphatic flow from the same approximate region in most species.[9]

Technique

Generally, the regional lymph node draining a specific body site is evaluated for MCT staging. A study evaluated the usefulness of complete staging in canine MCTs when there was no evidence of MCT spread to the local lymph node.[10] This study evaluated staging data from 220 dogs. The tumor distribution was based on the Patnaik system and included 24 grade 1, 152 grade 2, and 20 grade 3 MCTs. Some MCTs were additionally classified as having features of 2 grade categories. Some lymph nodes were not palpable or internal and not able to be sampled, leaving 119 dogs with sampled lymph nodes. Distant metastasis (spleen, liver, skin, or other lymph nodes) was detected in 15% whereas 31% had local lymph node metastasis. MCTs of the head were more likely to metastasize to the local lymph node and to distant sites. From this study it was determined that distant metastasis did not develop for dogs with a negative local lymph node. Of note, 42% of animals with lymph node metastasis did not develop distant spread or die as a result of the MCT. They also concluded thoracic radiography to have no value in the clinical staging of MCTs, although they may benefit the anesthetic evaluation and detection of comorbid conditions.

In the author's institution, the decision for full staging is usually based on tumor grade and/or lymph node status.

Often the decision regarding which lymph node to aspirate is based on assumption of drainage pattern. Information regarding lymph flow and lymph nodes likely to receive drainage from a given area can be found in anatomy texts; however, drainage in tumor-bearing animals may not reflect anatomic studies and may vary. Additionally, it may be challenging to predict the local lymph node for a given area, and a more accurate method of identification should be considered.

Lymphoscintigraphy involves intra- or peritumoral injection of radiopharmaceutical, allowing for detection of the lymph node(s) receiving lymph from the tumor. This is a relatively new area of investigation in veterinary medicine, although one report details its use.[11]

Outcomes

The utility of scintigraphy in MCT sentinel lymph node mapping was described by Worley in a series of 20 cases.[11] This study found 8 dogs to have sentinel lymph nodes that were different from the closest node and 12 dogs having metastasis. In all, 8 of 19 dogs needed additional treatment based on scintigraphy findings. This finding of unpredictable local lymph node detection is consistent with the author's clinical experience. We have found lymphoscintigraphy to be accurate, safe, cost effective and easy to perform. The author's approach has been to determine the sentinel lymph node by using scintigraphy, performing fine-needle aspiration, and basing additional staging tests on lymph node status. If cytology is equivocal or not diagnostic, the lymph node could be biopsied to determine its status, and biopsy could be done confidently knowing the location of the sentinel lymph node.

Surgical Treatment

Introduction

Surgical margins can be a complex concept, with the discussion not likely to be settled in this article. The most appropriate surgical margins or surgical dose used for MCTs is no exception to this challenging area of surgical oncology. The surgeon ultimately has to decide what is most appropriate for a given patient, client, budget, tumor, and location. Another feature of the tumor to consider is grade.

Outcomes—cutaneous mast cell tumors

Surgery cures far more MCTs than any other modality, and surgical excision should be considered the treatment of choice for most MCTs. Margin recommendations for MCTs vary depending on the source, but 2 to 3 cm lateral margins and 1 tissue plane deep (mesenchymal barrier) are frequently cited. In a study of 100 animals, 22% had grade 1 MCTs, 74% had grade 2% MCTs, and 4.3% had grade 3 MCTs.[12] All tumors evaluated had a mitotic index less than 5 per 10 high-power fields (hpf), which may be a limitation. Considering the 115 total tumors evaluated in this study, there were no local tumor recurrences when lateral margins greater than 1 cm and deep margins greater than 4 mm were removed. Consideration should be given to the study population, because few grade 3 MCTs and no grade 2 MCTs with mitotic indices greater than 5 per 10 hpf were in the study. Edema in the tissues and tumor demarcation were not correlated to outcome. Excessive edema formation from tumor manipulation or spontaneous cytokine release can make gross palpation and determination of tumor borders difficult.

Another study found histologically tumor-free margins in 29% of low-grade MCTs to be less than 3 mm with no local recurrences. In this same study, high-grade tumors were found to have a significant likelihood of local recurrence unrelated to the size of the surgical margin.[13]

An alternative to the one-size-fits-all approach to surgical margin for MCTs is adoption of a proportional margin approach. Instead of removing a set dimension of tissue, a proportional margin is determined based on the dimension of the individual tumor. The intent of this approach is to treat individual tumors with adequate margins without overtreating any neoplasms. Pratschke and colleagues[1] recently reported on the proportional margin technique; 40 dogs (47 tumors) were evaluated with both cutaneous (87%) and subcutaneous neoplasms (13%) included. Using the Patnaik system, 51% were grade 1, 44% were grade 2%, and 5% were grade 3. Using the 2-tiered system (described later), 90% were described as low grade and 10% described as high grade. The lateral surgical margin was based on the larger diameter of the mass (ie, a 2-cm tumor was removed with a 2-cm margin). The deep surgical margin included 1 fascial plane. The investigators included up to 4 cm of lateral margin for a 4 cm tumor, which is larger than the original intent of this approach (Dr Ralph Henderson, personal communication, 2012). Using this approach, the investigators reported 85% of tumors had histologically tumor-free margins. One dog with MCT was suspected to have recurrence and progressive disease. Few dogs received adjuvant treatment after incomplete excision.

Current controversies/future considerations

The question of how to best manage incompletely resected MCTs has come up often and is subject to debate. Local recurrence after incomplete resection is not a certainty. A substantial number of incompletely resected grade 2 MCTs never recur.[14] There is evidence that re-excision confers benefit to patients.[15] In a study of 64 dogs, 70 tumors were evaluated for the effect of additional local treatment, surgery, or radiation therapy (RT) compared with no additional treatment.[15] Survival times for re-excision (2930 days) and RT (2194 days) were significantly different from the group that did not receive any additional therapy (710 days). The re-excision group had a local recurrence rate of 13%. Local recurrence occurred in 8% of dogs that received RT and 38% for the group that received no additional local treatment.

There are several potential action plans to consider when faced with a biopsy report that indicates incomplete excision. Simple methods of investigation include fine-needle aspiration of the surgical site or scar to determine if any mast cells are present, which should be done carefully and methodically to ensure the entire surgical site is evaluated. An alternative to aspiration includes serial biopsies along the surgical site (eg, dermal biopsy punch), similarly to determine whether mast cells or residual MCT is present. Primary re-excision could also be considered depending on the ease of resection, location, available local tissues, patient vital reserves, and owner factors.

Outcomes—subcutaneous mast cell tumors

Subcutaneous MCTs are challenging to grade because the Patnaik system was developed for cutaneous neoplasms. Some investigators have considered MCTs originating in the subcutaneous fat to behave in a more malignant fashion than cutaneous neoplasms. A study evaluating 306 subcutaneous MCTs described their behavior.[16] Follow-up times were variable, with a mean of 848 days. More than 50% had follow-up times greater than 2 years. The MST was not reached and probability rates of survival at 6-month and 1-, 2-, and 5-year time points were 95%, 93%, 92%, and 86%, respectively. MCT-related deaths in this study were low (9%). Other important data from this study include tumor growth pattern with infiltrative tumors having approximately 3 times the likelihood of MCT-related mortality. Multinucleation, age at diagnosis, and mitotic index were prognostic. Mitotic index greater than 4 and other negative features were more life limiting (MST 140 days) than those with mitotic index less than 4 and lacking multinucleation and infiltrative growth (950 days). Metastasis was approximately 54 times more likely in dogs with mitotic index greater than 4 compared with those with a mitotic index of 0. Despite greater than 50% incomplete resections, 4% metastatic and 8% local recurrence rates suggest the prognosis for subcutaneous MCTs may be better than previously thought.

Nonsurgical management of mast cell tumors

Nonresectable MCTs are challenging to manage. Combinations of chemotherapy and RT may be considered. Tyrosine kinase inhibitors have become increasingly available and represent an additional treatment option in cases of nonresectable MCTs. The use of masitinib in 132 dogs with nonresectable tumors has been described.[17] Dogs with either recurrent or nonresectable grade 2 or grade 3 MCTs were assigned to treatment or control groups. Treatment with masitinib was significantly associated with time to progression of the disease and was independent of c-kit mutation status. Masitinib also improved the survival rate but not the MST. The median overall survival from this study was 617 days for the treatment group and 322 days for control. Survival to 24 months was predicted by tumor control at 6 months.

Another investigation of nonresectable grade 2 or 3 MCTs evaluated the use of paclitaxel.[18] Paclitaxel is a member of the taxane class of chemotherapeutics. Dogs (n = 252) were given paclitaxel or lomustine. Ultimately, lomustine was discontinued in 27 dogs due to development of hepatopathy. Three dogs in the paclitaxel group were discontinued for progression of disease or hepatopathy. A confirmed response at 2 weeks was 6.5 times more likely in the paclitaxel treatment group.

MAST CELL TUMORS IN CATS
Introduction

MCTs typically occur in the spleen, skin and intestine of cats.[19] In one report, splenic MCT was the reason for splenectomy in 53% of cats evaluated.[20] The head, neck, and trunk are common locations for cutaneous MCTs in cats. Surgical excision is the treatment of choice, and the outcome is not necessarily related to the surgical margins obtained.[19]

Outcome

Cutaneous MCTs in cats generally carry a favorable prognosis, with excision resulting in cure for the mastocytic forms.[19] Mastocytic MCTs are similar to canine MCTs. In a study evaluating CCNU chemotherapy of cats with cutaneous and visceral MCTs, the overall response rate to treatment was 50% (19/38) for a median duration of 168 days.[21] Overall MST for cats undergoing splenectomy has been reported.[20] Considering all causes of splenectomy (MCT, 53%; hemangiosarcoma, 21%; and lymphosarcoma, 11%). Considering all etiologies for splenectomy (MCT-53%, hemangiosarcoma-21% and lymphosarcoma-11%) the MST was reported as 197 days with the only significant factor being pre-operative weight loss. The MST for cats that experienced weight loss was 3 days versus those without weight loss of 293 days.

Histologic Grading Scheme for Mast Cell Tumors

Introduction

A 2-tiered grading scheme was proposed by Kiupel and colleagues[22] in 2011. As part of this study, a group of pathologists reviewed 95 cutaneous MCTs. Concordance among the pathologists using the Patnaik system was 75% for grade 3 tumors, 63% for grade 2 tumors, and 63% for grade 1 tumors. The 2-tiered system was evaluated because of inconsistent grading and lack of significant prognosis impact when stratifying grade 1 and grade 2 neoplasms. Criteria for high-grade MCTs include 1 or more of the items listed: 7 or more mitotic figures per 10 hpf, at least 3 multinucleated cells per 10 hpf, and at least 3 bizarre nuclei and karyomegaly. The 2-tiered system was shown to have 97% consistency and an association between high-grade MCTs and mortality/additional tumor development/metastasis and shorter survival times. The MST for low-grade MCTs was greater than 2 years, whereas the MST time for high-grade tumors was less than 4 months. The 2-tiered system was also shown a better predictor of survival compared with the Patnaik system, with the former having a 54 times hazard of death for high-grade tumors.

Outcome

The 2-tiered system was recently compared with the Patnaik system in a study of 137 MCTs.[23] The study aim was to determine whether either grading scheme could predict survival. For the Patnaik system, grade 3 MCTs had a worse prognosis, and no difference was found between grades 1 and 2 MCTs. Considering the Kiupel grading system, all Patnaik grade 1 MCTs were low grade and all Patnaik grade 3 MCTs were high grade; 86% of the grade 2 MCTs were low grade, and the remaining 14% were high grade. High-grade tumors resulted in a 1-year probability of survival of 46% whereas the low-grade 1-year probability of survival was 94%. The investigators concluded the 2-tiered system had prognostic value. They also mentioned that not all MCT behavior can be accurately predicted, because it is possible to see metastasis from a low-grade MCT.

SOFT TISSUE SARCOMAS
Introduction

Soft tissue sarcomas (STSs) are a diverse group of mesenchymal neoplasms with similar biologic behavior. The metastatic potential is typically low, especially for low- and intermediate-grade tumors. Several histologic tumor subtypes can be grouped under the STS heading, but this is not often necessary because their behavior is predictable.

Other types of sarcomas not included in the STS group include hemangiosarcoma, synovial cell sarcoma, and osteosarcoma.[24]

STSs are graded using a 3-tiered system composed of low, intermediate, and high grades. Features evaluated include differentiation, cellular features, mitotic index, and amount of necrosis.[24]

Staging

A diagnosis of STS can often be achieved with a fine-needle aspirate. Sometimes this is not possible because of poor cellular exfoliation. Histologic grade of an STS requires biopsy of the mass. An incisional biopsy may prove useful in planning definitive resection margins. Incisional biopsy also may help define the role of adjuvant therapy. If a clean margin is not expected based on tumor grade, number of prior surgeries, and location of the mass, such information should help surgeons and owners decide whether surgery would become the adjuvant in cases where RT is the primary treatment. Another scenario where incisional biopsy is useful is when considering an amputation where a low-grade neoplasm might be treated with more conservative margins.

Most sarcomas metastasize via blood to the lungs primarily; however, draining lymph nodes should be evaluated.[24] Metastasis is uncommon with STS and can be stratified according to tumor grade. Generally cited metastatic rates are less than 15% for low- to intermediate-grade STSs and up to 44% for high-grade STSs.[24]

Surgical Resection and Margin Considerations

Complete resection margins described for removal of STSs are variable but are often cited as 2 to 3 cm of normal tissue lateral to the mass and at least 1 fascial plane deep to the tumor.[24–26]

Certain locations are not amenable to tumor resections that include 3 cm of surrounding normal tissue. The limbs present a unique challenge where excision of significant skin often results in a wound that cannot be easily reconstructed. Immediate free skin grafting has been reported in 7 STS excisions.[27] The grafts were placed over beds of muscle and tendons, with no granulation tissue present. Superficial necrosis was evident on areas of 4 of the grafts and 3 had complete survival. Although this was a small number of cases, immediate grafting may be an option for reconstruction. A potential disadvantage of this strategy is performing reconstruction prior to receiving information about completeness of excision.

Resection of STS from the limbs without reconstruction has been reported.[25] To overcome the difficulties associated with 2- to 3-cm excisions, the investigators described second intention healing after excision of STS from the limbs in 31 dogs. Ten of these dogs were operated for prior incomplete resections and 21 were operated primarily. The STSs were removed with 2-cm lateral margins; the deep margin consisted of 1 fascial plane. The surgical sites were managed as open wounds covered by bandages during healing. The bandages were changed every 2 to 3 days until granulation tissue was visible, then weekly until epithelialization occurred.

For the animals that were operated for prior incomplete resections, 6 had histologically confirmed residual tumor. Low-grade tumors represented the majority (77%) of the STSs in this study, and none was high grade. The investigators reported the median time to healing for the wounds that closed completely (29/31) as 53 days. Two dogs were grafted because of delayed healing. This study reported no significant association between surface area of the wound related to the surface area of the patient and time to healing. Antimicrobial therapy was used in 4 dogs for presumed infections based on wound discharge character. Long-term complications were described for 26% of the dogs. Those complications included traumatic disruption of the healed epithelium and decreased range of motion secondary to contracture of the wounds after healing. One dog in this study was reported to have recurrence 560 days after surgery.

Open wound management after STS surgery resulted in local tumor control, but considerations regarding postoperative care exist. Owners electing a similar strategy should be well prepared for the amount of bandage care, frequency of bandage changes, cost, and time commitments. This strategy can be an attractive option for tumor resection because clear margins are expected to be achieved in most patients, but owner compliance and proper preparation for expected issues should be considered.

Another study evaluated STSs on the limbs of 35 dogs (37 tumors) for recurrence and disease-free interval after marginal excision (ie, working at or just outside the pseudocapsule)[28]; 11 of the tumors were palpably fixed and 26 were considered mobile. All tumors were considered low grade. Three tumors were recurrent after first opinion practice removal. The median size of the tumors in this study was 5 cm when measured at the tumor's longest dimension.

Analysis of the excision margins was possible in 35 of 37 STSs. They were considered incomplete in 12, clean but close in 12, and complete in 11. Four tumors (11%) had local recurrence, which was seen at 210, 450, 595, and 700 days after surgery. Recurrence occurred in the incomplete and clean but close groups but was not seen in the complete margin group. The mean survival time and disease-free interval were 704 days and 698 days, respectively. The results of this study highlight the importance of an incisional biopsy, and this approach may be an option in select situations with low-grade STSs.

Adjuvant Therapy for Soft Tissue Sarcomas

Introduction

Adjuvant therapy is generally considered for cases with incomplete STS resection. The decision-making process should take several things into account. Tumor grade, margin assessment, ease of additional surgery, risk of recurrence to the patient, patient health reserves, and owner factors are considerations. In general, options for incompletely resected STSs include frequent owner/primary care veterinarian surveillance, additional resection if feasible, amputation or body wall resection (if appropriate), RT, and/or metronomic chemotherapy.

Radiation therapy

RT is and has been an adjuvant treatment of incompletely resected STSs for some time. It is best in the setting of microscopic disease, therefore usually after excision or cytoreductive surgery. Postoperative RT has been reported to have a favorable outcome with 3-year survival rates greater than 80% and recurrence of STSs greater than 700 days.[26]

Marginal excision and coarse fractionated RT were evaluated in a study of 56 dogs.[26] RT was delivered to a total dose of 32 to 36 Gy in 4, 8- to 9-Gy fractions 7 days apart. In this study, 50 dogs received 4×8 Gy, 1 had 4×8.5 Gy, and 5 had 4×9 Gy. The investigators planned for 2- to 3-cm lateral margins and at least 1-cm deep margins of excision. Tumor grades were low in 33%, intermediate in 50%, and high in 17%. Histologically, resection margins were incomplete in all the cases. Complications observed during the RT treatment period were self-mutilation (1), partial wound dehiscence (1), and pathologic fracture of a metacarpal in the treatment field (1). Metastasis occurred in 9% and local recurrence in 18%. At the time of data collection, 75% of the dogs in the study were dead; of those, 35% had recurrence or metastasis. The estimated 1-, 3-, and 5-year recurrence rates were 19%, 30%, and 35%, respectively. An interesting finding from this study was that only the time from surgery to commencement of RT was a significant factor. The risk of recurrence was 8.6 times more likely in animals treated with RT within 1 month of surgery compared with treatment after 1 month. The 1-, 2-, and 3-year disease-free intervals from this study were 82%, 74%, and 70%, respectively.

Another study evaluated postoperative RT for incompletely resected STSs[29]; 37 dogs received 42 to 57 Gy administered in 3 to 4.2 Gy daily, Monday through Friday, fractions. The overall survival time was 1851 days, and the median time to recurrence was greater than 798 days. Oral STSs were also included in the data analysis of this article.

Chemotherapy

The administration of cytotoxic chemotherapy can be considered for dogs with STSs. Most clinicians reserve its use for high-grade tumors in which the risk of metastasis is greater compared with low and intermediate grades. Not all investigations support its use, however. A study evaluated the adjuvant use of doxorubicin in dogs with high-grade STSs[30]; 39 dogs were included and grouped as either surgery alone (n = 18) or surgery plus single-agent doxorubicin (n = 21). Overall disease-free period was 724 days, and the MST was 856 days. The administration of adjuvant chemotherapy did not have a significant effect on survival. Some considerations for this study include the variety of neoplasms described as STSs as well as the variable locations (some were visceral in origin).

Metronomic chemotherapy has been a significant shift in strategy from cytotoxic chemotherapy. Metronomic chemotherapy has been well described in the literature and is not exhaustively reviewed in this article. The metronomic administration of chemotherapy generally involves lower dose and increased frequency compared with traditional cytotoxic administration.[31] A critically important feature of metronomic chemotherapy is inhibition of angiogenesis. This is an important concept for the surgeon to understand because this strategy can have significant effects on the healing of surgical wounds. Timing of administration and discontinuation of metronomic chemotherapy should be considered when planning surgery.

Other effects of metronomic chemotherapy include immune system modification. This occurs because metronomic chemotherapy inhibits regulatory T-cell function.[31] Metronomic chemotherapy can involve coadministration of different drugs. For STSs, cyclophosphamide was evaluated.[31] Both regulatory T-cell numbers and blood vessel density of the tumors decreased in dogs with STSs treated with cyclophosphamide.

Additional evidence of metronomic chemotherapy effects in STSs has been described. A study reported on the clinical efficacy of metronomic cyclophosphamide and piroxicam.[32] Dogs with incompletely resected STSs were evaluated in 2 groups (treatment and control). A majority of the tumors evaluated in this study were intermediate grade. The disease-free interval for the treated compared with control groups was significantly different. Treated dogs did not reach the median whereas the median disease-free interval for the control group was 211 days. The statistically predicted disease-free interval in the treatment group was 410 days. When controlling for surgeon characteristics, the treated group had a significant difference compared with the control group for tumors of the extremities. Tumors of the trunk had similar findings. Adverse reactions to the drugs in the protocol occurred in 40% of the treated dogs, although they were usually mild. Sterile hemorrhagic cystitis developed in 3 of 30 dogs. Changing the dosing interval from daily to every other day managed most of the adverse events. These studies highlight the importance of metronomic administration of chemotherapy in dogs with STSs. More investigation into the mechanisms of action is ongoing and will likely change as understanding of their use increases.

Current Controversies/Future Considerations

Incomplete surgical margins in dogs with STSs can be handled in several ways. As described previously, options include re-excision, surgery followed by RT, surgery followed by metronomic chemotherapy, surgery followed by diligent surveillance with plan for re-excision or other adjuvant if needed, and combinations of these options. Knowing what to do with each patient on receipt of the pathology report can be challenging. Each case likely needs to be considered individually with the pet and owner in mind.

Re-excision of the surgical wound with a margin of normal tissue has been reported to have a recurrence rate of 15%.[32,33] Another study evaluated STSs managed by primary care veterinarians.[34] Questionnaires were used to evaluate clinical findings and outcome in 350 cases. Unplanned surgeries were common, with only 4% having a histologic diagnosis and 17% having a cytologic diagnosis before surgical excision.

The MST was not reached with a 5-year survival of 70%. Extent of the surgical excision was not associated with survival or recurrence of the STS. Local recurrence occurred in 21% of the cases. High-grade STSs were significantly associated with recurrence of the mass.

FELINE INJECTION SITE SARCOMAS
Introduction

Injection site sarcomas represent a significant challenge to veterinary surgeons and cat and pet owners. These are often deeply invasive masses that do not respect mesenchymal barriers, allowing them to invade surrounding tissues. A variety of treatments have been used, and injection site sarcomas are often a model example of the need for multimodal therapy. Tumor recurrence is a significant problem (up to 69%) whereas metastasis is not as common, generally less than 20%.[24,35–37]

Surgical Therapy

A recent report evaluated surgery alone as a treatment of cats with injection site sarcomas.[35] Lateral surgical margins were described as 5 cm from the tumor edge or scar; deep margins were 2 muscle planes or bone deep to the tumor. Deep margins included chest and abdominal wall, dorsal spinous processes, ilial wing, and scapula.

In this study, 91 cats were evaluated. The median maximal tumor diameter reported was 4 cm. Complete resection margins were reported in 97% of the cases. Local tumor recurrence was reported in 14% of the cases; most were from high-grade sarcomas. The overall MST was 901 days, and 20% of the cats developed metastasis. MST for cats with recurrence was 499 days, and 1461 days for those cats without recurrence. Metastasis and local recurrence were determined to be predictive of survival. Incisional dehiscence was the most common major complication reported. Minor complications were uncommon.

Ancillary Therapy

RT is frequently used in the management of injection site sarcomas in cats. A study evaluated cats with STSs and the effect of RT timing as neoadjuvant or adjuvant treatment after surgical excision.[38] The investigators retrospectively evaluated 79 cats, 55 of which were treated with surgery prior to RT; 24 cats had incisional biopsies followed by RT and surgery. Mild to moderate anemia was observed in 71% of cats. The MST for all cats was 520 days, with 1- and 2-year survival rates of 62% and 42%, respectively. Factors found significant for survival included anemia and the timing of RT relative to surgery. The MST for cats treated with neoadjuvant RT was 310 days compared with 705 days for those cats receiving RT after surgery. A selection bias toward larger, more difficult to remove tumors may occur when considering neoadjuvant RT.

NOVEL IMAGING SYSTEMS

A novel, wide field-of-view imaging system coupled with a near-infrared fluorescent probe has been described for real-time excision margin assessment in dogs.[39] The dogs were given an injection of cathepsin-activated near-infrared imaging probe prior to surgery and no adverse events relative to probe injection were identified. In 9 of 10 tumors, the histologic assessment of margins correlated with the operative imaging findings.

This is a major advancement toward the development of a point-of-care instrument capable of determining a tumor-free operative site. Additional studies with equipment like this should help determine its role in veterinary surgery. This type of imaging may have a significant role in veterinary surgical oncology in the future.

REFERENCES

1. Pratschke KM, Atherton MJ, Sillito JA, et al. Evaluation of a modified proportional margins approach for surgical resection of mast cell tumors in dogs: 40 cases (2008–2012). J Am Vet Med Assoc 2013;243:1436–41.
2. Cohen D, Reif JS, Brodey RS, et al. Epidemiological analysis of the most prevalent sites and types of canine neoplasia observed in a veterinary hospital. Cancer Res 1974;34:2859–68.
3. Dorn CR, Taylor DO, Schneider R, et al. Survey of animal neoplasms in Alameda and Contra Costa Counties, California. II. Caner morbidity in dogs and cats from Alameda County. J Natl Cancer Inst 1968;40:307–18.
4. Kelsey JL, Moore AS, Glickman LT. Epidemiological studies of risk factors for cancer in pet dogs. Epidemiol Rev 1998;20:204–17.
5. Book AP, Fidel J, Wills T. Correlation of ultrasound findings, liver and spleen cytology and prognosis in the clinical staging of high metastatic risk canine mast cell tumors. Vet Radiol Ultrasound 2011;52:548–54.
6. Hume CT, Kiupel M, Rigatti L, et al. Outcomes of dogs with grade 3 mast cell tumors: 43 cases (1997–2007). J Am Anim Hosp Assoc 2011;47:37–44.
7. Stefanello D, Valenti P, Faverzani S. Ultrasound-guided cytology of the spleen and liver: a prognostic tool in canine cutaneous mast cell tumor. J Vet Intern Med 2009;23:1051–7.
8. Marconato L, Bettini G, Giacoboni G, et al. Clinicopathological features and outcome for dogs with mast cell tumors and bone marrow involvement. J Vet Intern Med 2008;22:1001–7.
9. Bezuidenhout AJ. The lymphatic system. In: Evans HE, editor. Miller's anatomy of the dog. 3rd edition. Toronto: WB Saunders; 1993. p. 717–57.
10. Warland J, Fuster-Amores I, Newbury W, et al. The utility of staging in canine mast cell tumours. Vet Comp Oncol 2014;12(4):287–98.
11. Worley DR. Incorporation of sentinel lymph node mapping in dogs with mast cell tumors: 20 consecutive procedures. Vet Comp Oncol 2014;12:215–26.
12. Schultheiss PC, Gardiner DW, Rao S, et al. Association of tumor characteristics and size of surgical margins with clinical outcome after surgical removal of cutaneous mast cell tumors in dogs. J Am Vet Med Assoc 2011;232:1464–9.
13. Donnelly L, Mullin C, Balko J, et al. Evaluation of histological grade and histologically tumour-free margins as predictors of local recurrence in completely excised canine mast cell tumours. Vet Comp Oncol 2015;13:70–6.
14. Seguin B, Leibman NF, Bregazzi VS, et al. Recurrence rate, clinical outcome and cellular proliferation indices as prognostic indicators after incomplete surgical excision of cutaneous grade II mast cell tumors: 28 dogs (1994–2002). J Vet Intern Med 2006;20:933–40.
15. Kry KL, Boston SE. Additional local therapy with primary re-excision or radiation therapy imporves survival and local control after incomplete or close surgical excision of mast cell tumors in dogs. Vet Surg 2014;43:182–9.
16. Thompson JJ, Pearl DL, Yager JA, et al. Canine subcutaneous mast cell tumor characterization and prognostic indices. Vet Pathol 2011;48:156–68.
17. Hahn KA, Legendre AM, Shaw NG, et al. Evaluation of 12- and 24-month survival rates after treatment with masitinib in dogs with nonresectable mast cell tumors. Am J Vet Res 2010;71:1354–61.

18. Vail DM, von Euler AW, Rusk L, et al. A randomized trial investigating the efficacy and safety of water soluble micellar paclitaxel for treatment of nonresectable grade 2 or 3 mast cell tumors in dogs. J Vet Intern Med 2012;26:598–607.
19. Henry C, Herrera C. Mast cell tumors in cats clinical update and possible new treatment avenues. J Feline Med Surg 2013;15:41–7.
20. Gordon SS, McClaran JK, Bergman PJ, et al. Outcome following splenectomy in cats. J Feline Med Surg 2010;12:256–61.
21. Rassnick KM, Williams LE, Kristal O, et al. Lomustine for the treatment of mast cell tumors in cats: 38 cases (1999–2005). J Am Vet Med Assoc 2008;232:1200–5.
22. Kiupel M, Webster KL, Bailey S, et al. Proposal of a 2 –tier histologic grading system for canine cutaneous mast cell tumors to more accurately predict biological behavior. Vet Pathol 2011;48:147–55.
23. Sabattini S, Scarpa F, Berlato D, et al. Histologic grading of canine mast cell tumor: is 2 better than 3? Vet Pathol 2015;52(1):70–3.
24. Van Nimwegen S, Kirpensteijn J. Specific disorders. In: Tobias KM, Johnston SA, editors. Veterinary surgery small animal. St Louis (MO): Elsevier; 2012. p. 1303–39.
25. Prpich CY, Santamaria AC, Simcock JO, et al. Second intention healing after wide local excision of soft tissue sarcomas in the distal aspects of the limbs in dogs: 31 cases (2005–2012). J Am Vet Med Assoc 2014;244:187–94.
26. Demetriou JL, Brearley MJ, Constantino-Casas F, et al. Intential marginal excision of canine limb soft tissue sarcomas followed by radiotherapy. J Small Anim Pract 2012;53:174–81.
27. Tong T, Simpson DJ. Free Skin grafts for immediate wound coverage following tumour resection from the canine distal limb. J Small Anim Pract 2012;53:520–5.
28. Stefanello D, Marello E, Roccabiaanca P, et al. Marginal excision of low-grade spindle cell sarcoma of canine extremities. Vet Surg 2008;37:462–5.
29. Forrest LJ, Chun R, Adams WM, et al. Postoperative radiotherapy for canine soft tissue sarcomas. J Vet Intern Med 2000;14:578–82.
30. Selting KA, Powers BE, Thompson LJ, et al. Outcome of dogs with high grade soft tissue sarcomas treated with and without adjuvant doxorubicin chemotherapy: 39 cases (1996–2004). J Am Vet Med Assoc 2005;227:1442–8.
31. Burton JH, Mitchell L, Thamm DH, et al. Low dose cyclophosphamide selectively decreases regulatory t cells and inhibits angiogenesis in dogs with soft tissue sarcomas. J Vet Intern Med 2011;25:920–6.
32. Elmslie RE, Glawe P, Dow SW. Metronomic therapy with cyclophosphamide and piroxicam effectively delays tumor recurrence in dogs with incompletely resected soft tissue sarcomas. J Vet Intern Med 2008;22:1373–9.
33. Bacon NJ, Dernell WS, Ehrhart N, et al. Evaluation of primary re-excision after recent inadequate resection of soft tissue sarcomas in dogs: 41 cases (1999–2004). J Am Vet Med Assoc 2007;230:548–54.
34. Bray JP, Polton GA, McSorran KD, et al. Canine soft tissue sarcomas managed in fist opinion practice: outcome in 350 cases. Vet Surg 2014;43(7):774–82.
35. Phelps HA, Kuntz CA, Milner RJ, et al. Radical excision with five-centimeter margins for treatment of feline injection-site sarcomas: 91 cases (1998–2002). J Am Vet Med Assoc 2011;239:97–106.
36. Giudice C, Stefanello D, Sala M, et al. Feline injection-site sarcoma: recurrence, tumor grading and surgical margin status evaluated using the three-dimensional histological technique. Vet J 2010;186:84–8.
37. Cronin K, Page RL, Spodnick G, et al. Radiation therapy and surgery for fibrosarcoma in 33 cats. Vet Radiol Ultrasound 1998;39:51–6.

38. Mayer MN, Treuil PL, LaRue SM. Radiotherapy and surgery for feline soft tissue sarcoma. Vet Radiol Ultrasound 2009;50:669–72.
39. Eward WC, Mito JK, Eward CA, et al. A novel imaging system permits real-time in vivo tumor bed assessment after resection of naturally occurring sarcomas in dogs. Clin Orthop Relat Res 2013;471:834–42.

Facilitation of Soft Tissue Surgery

Surgical Staplers and Vessel Sealing Devices

Laura E. Peycke, DVM, MS

KEYWORDS

- Stapling • Vascular sealing • Vessel sealing devices • Endoscopic staplers
- Endoscopic vessel sealing devices • Surgical devices • Mechanical hemostasis

KEY POINTS

- Medical surgical devices have improved efficiency of surgery without compromising confidence in hemorrhage control.
- Surgical stapling instruments can decrease tissue trauma, contamination, and the anesthetic period in multiple body systems, including gastrointestinal, urogenital, cardiovascular, pulmonary, and skin.
- Vascular sealing devices can coagulate vessels and hemorrhagic tissues effectively and quickly.
- When used within recommended guidelines, vascular sealing devices are reported to reduce surgical time and provide occlusion sufficient to counteract arterial pressures without using foreign material.
- Endoscopic stapling and vessel sealing devices follow similar concepts as conventional surgical staplers and vascular sealing devices, but are designed to be used with laparoscopic and thoracoscopic procedures.

INTRODUCTION

Recent advances and acceptance of various medical devices have clearly helped in the efficiency, simplicity, and effectiveness of veterinary surgery. The goals of surgery include efficient methods and minimal surgical times, delicate tissue handling techniques, confidence with tissue reconstruction, and minimizing contamination, leakage and complications. Mechanical means of suturing, cutting, and hemostasis assist with accomplishing these goals. Most recently, stapling instrumentation and vascular sealing devices have become common instruments on all levels of surgery because of their ease of use and increase in surgical efficiency.

The author has nothing to disclose.
Department of Veterinary Small Animal Clinical Sciences, College of Veterinary Medicine and Biomedical Sciences, Texas A&M University, 422 Raymond Stotzer Parkway, College Station, TX 77845, USA
E-mail address: lpeycke@cvm.tamu.edu

Vet Clin Small Anim 45 (2015) 451–461
http://dx.doi.org/10.1016/j.cvsm.2015.01.010
0195-5616/15/$ – see front matter © 2015 Elsevier Inc. All rights reserved.

STAPLING INSTRUMENTS

Surgical stapling methods have been explored widely and used in veterinary surgery. Relationships between surgical goals and their use have been shown and their development has been enhanced by modifications for ease of use in veterinary surgery.[1] By the early 1980s, the use of stapling instrumentation was being recognized and used in the United States based on clinical studies and greater availability.[2]

The use of surgical stapling requires the knowledge of use for each stapling device. In no situation, however, should the use of a stapler compensate for poor surgical practice. Attention to principles of soft tissue surgery (Halstead's principles), as well as proper use of each surgical stapler must be followed to ensure surgical success. Principles that have been reported include[3]:

1. Do not staple tissues that are inflamed, edematous, or lack a vascular supply.
2. Every staple must penetrate all tissue layers.
3. Staple size should be accurate; tissues should not be too thick to be penetrated or too thin to support the staple.
4. Tissues should be inspected thoroughly before stapler application to ensure proper alignment and no capturing of inadvertent tissues.
5. Stapling devices should be removed carefully to avoid disrupting the staples.
6. Tissues should be grasped gently before removal of the stapler to check for hemorrhage, leakage, or loose staples.

Conventional Stapling Devices

Thoracoabdominal stapler

The thoracoabdominal (TA) stapler is a versatile stapler that applies staggered rows of B-shaped, titanium or stainless steel staples into tissue or across vascular pedicles.[4] The instrument consists of a handle with a handle and trigger configuration and a "U-shaped" end that accepts the vascular tissues or pedicle to be ligated. The noncrushing nature of the B-shaped staples allows for normal capillary blood flow between the staggered rows of staples, but adequately provides hemostasis at the border of excised tissues or vascular structures.[5] Reusable and disposable TA staplers are available and come in various widths for multiple tissue types. Reusable TA staple instruments have staple cartridge widths that are color-coded and are available in 30 mm (white), 55 mm (blue), and 90 mm (green). Disposable staplers come in 30, 45, 60, and 90 mm widths. Decisions on which staple size to use depend on confidence with compression of tissues and vessels with the size of staples selected. Exceeding the width of the pedicle or tissue is a better decision than stopping short of the tissue edge.[6] White cartridges (also known as V3), are only available in 30 mm widths and apply 3 rows of staples 3.0 mm wide by 2.5 mm in length and compress to a height of 1.0 mm.[4–6] Blue cartridges are available in 55 and 90 mm widths and apply 2 rows of staples that are 4.0 mm wide by 3.5 mm in length and compress to a height of 1.5 mm.[4–6] Green cartridges are available in 55 and 90 mm widths and apply 2 rows of staples that are 4.0 mm wide by 4.8 mm in length and compress to a height of 2.0 mm.[4–6]

Tissues are inserted through the anvils of the staple cartridge and secured when the approximating lever is closed. At this point, alignment is checked and adjustments made by releasing the approximating lever and realigning the tissues, if necessary. Excessive force should not be necessary to close the approximating lever and the retaining pin should engage to ensure appropriate compression of tissues. The safety is released and the trigger is squeezed to apply the staples across the tissue.[4,5] Before releasing the stapled tissues, the instrument can be used as a guide for cutting. Upon tissue release, grasping and inspecting tissues for hemostasis and thorough compression should be done.

TA staplers have been used in countless body system tissues; however, the most commonly reported tissues include gastrointestinal (esophageal resection, Billroth procedures, intestinal anastomosis and closure, typhlectomy, rectal tear closure, rectal tumor removal, and closure of the intestinal ends in the final stage of a gastrointestinal intestinal anastomosis [GIA] stapled procedure), endocrine (pancreatectomy), respiratory (partial or complete lung lobectomy), lymphatic organs (splenectomy), reproductive tissues (ovarian, vaginal and uterine stump closure; partial prostatectomy), urinary system (bladder closure, nephrectomy), and cardiovascular (right atrial appendage tumors).[5–19] Recent results suggest that the TA stapler is an efficient and safe method of vascular occlusion and tumor resection. Despite the need for further ancillary occlusion methods in some cases, its use is becoming the standard of care for many procedures in dogs and cats.[20–24] Advantages include significant decreases in operative time, decreased hemorrhage and necrosis of tissues. Disadvantages include incomplete ligation of vascular tissue, decrease in lumen size, leakage of air or fluid, and technical errors (**Table 1**).[5,20,22,25]

Gastrointestinal anastomosis and intestinal linear anastomosis staplers

The GIA stapler is a linear stapling instrument that consists of 2 interlocking halves that form a flat handle with 2 straight limbs.[26] One-half of the instrument holds a stapling cartridge that delivers 4 rows of B-shaped titanium staples and the other half holds an anvil.[4,5] Typically, the device has an embedded cutting blade that divides the tissue between the second and third row of staples.[4–6] The reusable form of this instrument comes in lengths of 50 and 90 mm and accepts stapling cartridges that deliver 4.0 mm wide B-shaped staples that begin at a height of 3.8 mm and compress to a final height of 1.5 mm.[4,5] Disposable staplers come in a variety of lengths (50, 60, 80, and 90 mm) and have color-coded cartridges (green and blue) that deliver B-shaped staples

Table 1			
Thoracoabdominal (TA) staple dimensions of specific reusable staple cartridges			
Instrument and Cartridge	**Staple (Top) Width by (Arm) Length (mm)**	**Closed Staple Height (mm)**	**Indications**
TA 30 (V3): white	3.0 × 2.5	1.0	Large vascular pedicle Right atrial appendage tumor Lung lobectomy
TA 30, 55, 90: blue	4.0 × 3.5	1.5	Partial lung lobectomy Uterine stump Typhlectomy Liver lobectomy Esophageal resection Paraprostatic cysts Partial prostatectomy Enterotomy closure Partial splenectomy
TA 30, 55, 90: green	4.0 × 4.8	2.0	Liver lobectomy Paraprostatic cysts Partial prostatectomy Gastrotomy closure Partial splenectomy

4.0 mm in width. The difference between cartridges is the green cartridge has an initial height of 4.8 mm and compresses to 2.0 mm, and the blue cartridge has an initial height of 3.8 mm and compresses to 1.5 mm in height (**Table 2**).[5]

With the reusable GIA stapler, the halves of the stapler are separated using the lock lever to load the stapling cartridge. The flexibility of this instrument allows for individual introduction of the halves into a lumen, such as bowel, or on the either side of tissue to be resected, such as liver or lung.[7–9] To use the GIA instrument, the instrument is positioned over the tissue segments and the back end of the stapler is aligned and compressed by closing the locking lever. Once inspection of the tissue to be resected or anastomosed is satisfactory, the push bar tab between the handles is slid toward the jaws to apply the staples and cut between them with a blade. The incision made by the bisecting blade stops 8.0 mm before crossing the end of the staple line. The staples should penetrate the entire thickness of tissues and inspection of these tissues should be performed at this point.[4] If used on the bowel in a side-by-side manner, the result will be a linear opening between 2 bowel segments. The remaining open edges of intestinal tissue should be closed using hand sutures or a TA stapler.[5] Indications for this stapling instrument include partial gastrectomy, pyloroplasy, typhlectomy, gastropexy, cholecystoenterostomy, prostatic cyst resection, lung lobectomy, liver lobectomy, esophageal and rectal diverticulum removal, and rectal polyp resection.[4–15,26,27] Use of the stapler with these indications requires slight modifications in technique and should be reviewed before use.

Reported advantages include decreased tissue manipulation, immediate increase in bursting strength, superior strength in lag-phase of healing and reduced inflammation and necrosis.[5,28,29] Complications associated with the use of the GIA stapler include intestinal leakage and abscess formation; however, the relevance and application of reported results have been variable and questioned.[5,28,29] Prevention of these complications has been attributed to leakage at the interface of the GIA and TA staple lines and within the staple line of the GIA stapler where the anastomotic "crotch" forms. Reinforcement with hand sutures at these sites has been recommended; however, recent studies have suggested that the incidence of leakage was greater at the GIA and TA staple intersection and off-setting the instruments so the staple lines are not directly across from each other when the TA stapler is applied may assist with prevention of leakage.[7,28,29] The relatively low complication rate reported in multiple studies supporting the use of the GIA stapler in functional end-to-end anastomosis, even in the hands of surgeons with limited exposure to the instrument, supports that it is a safe, efficient, and reliable method for intestinal closure.[5,7,28,29]

End-to-end anastomotic staplers

End-to-end anastomotic (EEA) staplers are tubular instruments that apply a circumferential double row of staples.[4] The result of this staple configuration is a double row of B-shaped, titanium staples that create a double layer inverting anastomosis of tissues of the alimentary canal.[4,5] The 2-piece instrument consists of a dome-shaped anvil and a long tubular portion that holds the staple cartridge.[5] The cartridges of the stapler have an outer diameter of 31, 28, and 25 mm and produce an anastomosis inner

Table 2			
Gastrointestinal intestinal anastomosis dimensions			
Staple Cartridge	**Staple Width (mm)**	**Open Height (mm)**	**Closed Height (mm)**
Blue	3.0	3.8	1.5
Green	3.0	4.8	2.0

diameter of 21, 18, and 15 mm.[4] The staples have a width of 4.0 mm and a height of 4.8 mm and compress to a height of 2.0 mm.[4] Disposable EEA instruments are available in similar and smaller sizes for use in smaller dogs and cats (**Table 3**).[4]

Ovoid-shaped sizers are equal to the outer staple cartridge diameter and are used to determine appropriate sizing.[5] Use of lubrication can assist with insertion of the sizer. The ovoid sizers may also be used to facilitate insertion of the stapler.[4] End-to-end staplers may be used for end-to-end anastomosis in the gastrointestinal tract. Introduction of the stapler can be made through the anus or through a purposely created orifice adjacent to the desired anastomotic location (via celiotomy). Anastomotic tissue ends are secured to the central rod portion of the stapler with a full-thickness pursestring suture. The application of this pursestring suture may be placed manually or facilitated by using a Furniss pursestring device.[4] The tissue ends are brought together along the central rod and the pursestring sutures are tightened between the anvil and staple cartridge. Careful inspection should be done to ensure that the intestinal tissue edges are inverted and aligned. The unit is then compressed by tightening the wing nut and the handle is squeezed to apply the staples. An embedded circular blade concurrently incises the pursestring sutures and redundant tissue away from the inverted portion of the tissue.[4,5] Once the stapler is removed, the doughnut-shaped excised tissues are removed and inspected to determine that the staples penetrated the full thickness of the tissues.[4] If an enterotomy has been created for instrument insertion, it should be closed manually or with a TA stapler.[4–6] Common locations and indications for usage of the EEA stapler in small animal surgery include colorectal/colonic, esophageal, and end-to-side gastroduodenostomy and gastroesophageal surgeries.[4,7,10,15–18]

Ligate-divide staple stapler

The ligate-divide staple (LDS) device has a handle and trigger that is used to apply simultaneously 2 titanium vascular clips to a vessel and cut between stapled tissues automatically after the clips have been applied. The staples are U-shaped and form crescent-shaped staples once compressed. They come in a regular size (5.79 mm wide × 5.23 mm tall open and a closure width of 5.33 mm wide, staples placed 6.35 mm apart) and wide size (8.0 mm wide × 7.2 mm tall and a closure width of 7.3 mm, staples placed 9.53 mm apart; **Table 4**).[5,13] The advantages of the LDS include ease of use, speed of application, and in procedures where multiple vessels require ligation, such as splenectomies.[13,14] Disadvantages include increased expense and lack of security when compared with other methods of vascular occlusion.[13,19] Other reported specific indications for its use include ovariohysterectomy, ligation and division of a patent ductus arteriosus or ligamentum arteriosus, and ligation of pulmonary vasculature during pneumonectomy.[30,31] This device should not be used on vessels that cannot be compressed to a thickness of 0.75 mm and a width of 7.0 mm.[13]

Table 3
End-to-end anastomotic dimensions

Cartridge Outer Diameter (mm)	Cartridge Inner Diameter (Knife Diameter; mm)	Staple Width (mm)	Open Staple Height (mm)	Closed Staple Height (mm)
25	15.0	4.0	4.8	2.0
28	18.0	4.0	4.8	2.0
31	21.2	4.0	4.8	2.0

Table 4			
Ligate-divide staple (LDS) dimensions			
LDS Type	Staple Width (Open), mm	Staple Height (mm)	Staple Width (Closed), mm
Regular	5.79	5.23	5.33
Wide	8.0	7.2	7.3

Vascular clips

Vascular clips are individual hemostatic V-shaped staples that can be applied quickly and accurately in areas that are difficult to reach. Application of the staples can be done with a single-clip applicator or with an automatic instrument loaded with multiple staples. These clips are an alternative to individual ligatures for small vessels and may serve as a radiopaque boundary to a surgical area or tumor excision.[5,13] They are most commonly composed of stainless steel, titanium, or an absorbable material. A variety of clip lengths are available; however, regardless of the manufacturer notations, the vessel size should fill only one-third to two-thirds of the length of the clip.[19,32] To prevent slippage and failure of the clip, the vessels or tissues to be clipped should have enough tissue to allow the clips to sit at least 2 to 3 mm from the edge of the excision. These clips are most useful in situations where surgical exposure and access is limited by surrounding structures, multiple small vessels require ligation and the vascular clips are as efficacious as suture ligatures. Disadvantages include decreased security in vessel occlusion.[19] The most common indications reported include laparoscopic and thoracoscopic application and as a novel technique for ligation of a patent ductus arteriosus.[9,13,14,33,34] After application, care should be taken to avoid dislodging the clip from the end of the vessel.[5,13]

Skin staplers

Surgical skin staples are used to accurately oppose tissue edges after tissue incision or trauma. Skin staples have a straight cross member with 2 shorter legs. Upon firing of the instrument, the cross member lies flat across the tissue to be opposed, the tissue is penetrated, and the legs are brought together to form an incomplete rectangular shape that is slightly smaller than its original width.[5] Typically, surgical skin staples are made of 316L stainless steel and are available in regular (4.8–6.1 mm width) and wide sizes (6.5–7.0 mm width) and have a wire diameter of just greater than 0.5 mm.[35] The staple leg length is variable, but the wide staples have longer legs, which may be beneficial in edematous tissue, but a disadvantage if deep tissue penetration by the staples is not desired.[35] Staples should be placed 0.5 to 1.0 cm apart.

Advantages to skin staple use include increased speed of tissue closure and subsequent cost effectiveness. Disadvantages are associated with incorrect application that results in poor tissue apposition, decreased wound security, staple disruption before healing, and eversion of wound edges. Many of these disadvantages can be avoided with proper soft tissue principles, such as absence of tension on the wound edges and use of thumb forceps to assist with accurate staple placement.

Use in animals has revealed variable results, with the most recent results suggesting use of skin staples as a risk factor for postoperative infection at the surgical site.[36,37] In 1 recent study, the use of surgical staples in dogs undergoing stifle surgery significantly increased the risk of postoperative inflammation–infection to 9.1% (21/231) when compared with wounds closed with nonmetallic suture (5.1% [34/671]).[36] Therefore, it was concluded that the odds of developing surgical site inflammation–infection was 1.9 times higher when stainless steel staples were used for skin closure, when compared with other methods. It was theorized that the reason for the increase in inflammation–infection at the surgical site could be attributed to the noncompliant nature of metal staples and increase in tissue irritation that could result in additional inflammation and subsequent self-trauma. To avoid these side effects, a recommendation of a minimum distance of 4.0 to 6.5 mm between the staple cross bar and the tissue should be maintained.[36]

Indications for the use of surgical skin staples include primary wound closure; securing skin grafts, tubes, and wound dressings; enterotomy and gastrotomy closure; small intestinal resection; and anastomosis and gastropexy.[35,38–40] Experimentally, equal bursting strength, lumen diameter, and circumference and healing characteristics were reported with the use of skin staples when compared with hand-sewn techniques.[39] Clinically, limited case reports suggest that staples are approximately 3 times faster and can be used effectively with closure of enterotomy sites and in the cases of resection and anastomosis.[38]

Although ease, precision, and a decrease in surgical time are benefits of skin stapler use, the manufacturer's recommendations should be consulted before use of the stapler.[35] Removal of skin staples should be done with a staple extractor instrument, which spreads the staple arms for easier removal from the skin.

Endoscopic Stapling Devices

With the recent advances in minimally invasive procedures, stapling equipment designed specifically for laparoscopic procedures has been developed and adapted for veterinary surgery. Thoracoscopic and laparoscopic procedures provide a magnified view and increased visualization of vital structures. With advances in these procedures and the improvement of minimally invasive stapling and vascular sealing instrumentation, vascular structures can be occluded confidently and diseased tissues can be removed safely.[41] Most endoscopic stapling instruments have an articulating head and use staple cartridges that simultaneously place 6 rows of staples. An embedded cutting blade incises through the middle of the stapled line, leaving 3 rows of staples on each side and providing a seal to each sides of the excised tissues. EndoGIA stapling cartridges (Covidien, Norwalk, CT) are able to deliver 30, 45, and 60 mm length staples. The staple leg lengths are available in sizes of 2.0, 2.5, 3.5, and 4.8 mm. Of these cartridges, the 30 and 60 mm length staples have 3.5 mm leg length. Many open and minimally invasive procedures using EndoGIA staples have been described and include lung lobectomy,[42] right auricular mass removal,[43] and other procedures to remove diseased tissues and provide vessel occlusion.

VESSEL SEALING DEVICES

As an alternative to ligatures and stapling instruments, vessel sealing devices have been developed to provide hemostasis effectively to vascular tissues in open and minimally invasive procedures.[22,44,45] These devices use electrothermal bipolar electrosurgery energy and pressure to induce denaturing and fusion of collagen and elastin within the vessel wall and surrounding tissues for vascular occlusion.[46] A thrombus proximal to the sealing site also contributes to occlusion of the vasculature.[44] The LigaSure system (Covidien, Inc, Mansfield, MA) is available as a standalone unit or in combination with other electrosurgery functions (ForceTriad, Covidien). The LigaSure utilizes a generator attached to a variety of handheld instruments with jaws designed to deliver bipolar energy into the grasped tissues. This system generator measures the electrical impedance (density) of the tissues and a precise amount of bipolar radiofrequency energy is generated. When combined with pressure within the jaws of the instrument, a calculated amount of energy is introduced to the tissues. The sensing of tissue impedance within the jaws of the instrument is able to measure and adjust energy from the generator, thereby ensuring an effective seal. Once feedback from the instrument to the generator is acknowledged and adequate levels for occlusion have been reached, an audible tone is heard and the cycle is complete. If the instrument is being used properly, the operator should be confident that a permanent seal has been created with minimal thermal damage of up to 2 mm in the surrounding tissue.[44,46] The device is approved for vessels measuring 7 mm in diameter or smaller; however, when using the instrument for tissue dissection, larger bundles can be grasped and effectively sealed.[46]

Although the LigaSure device is a very commonly used vessel sealing device, other units have also become available in the marketplace. The SurgRx EnSeal device (Ethicon, Cincinnati, OH) also relies on bipolar energy to seal vessels to 7 mm in diameter, but seems to control thermal spread and tissue damage to 1 mm by limiting the tissue temperature to 100°C.[46] This system limits unwanted thermal effect with high compression jaw force and precise control of energy to the tissues at the jaw-tissue interface.[46] The Harmonic system (Ethicon Endo-surgery) is another option for coagulation and cutting of tissues with delivery of ultrasonic waves at about 55,000 vibrations per second (55.5 kHz) to seal vessels up to 5 mm in diameter. With the use of high-frequency vibrations, lower temperatures (ranging from 50° to 100°C) are produced and applied to form an "oscillating saw" effect to cut tissues and denature proteins to seal vessels.[46]

The use of vessel sealing devices has improved the quality of surgical procedures with its efficiency, effectiveness, and ease of use.[46] Human and veterinary studies have made comparisons between units and also examined their use on tissues other than vessels.[47] Studies to examine the effectiveness and speed of these devices in procedures, collateral damage to tissue, blood loss, and use in minimally invasive surgery have been done and support their use in veterinary surgery.[22,40,45,46,48-52] Benefits that have been noted include efficient and complete hemostasis of vessels, adequate arterial bursting pressure, absence of foreign material, and no need for additional ligation support.[44] In a study by Rivier and Monnet,[44] it was determined that use of a vessel sealant device (Ligasure) provided adequate hemostasis and would provide adequate resistance to blood pressure in splenectomies when the splenic vessel and other associated vessels were isolated and coagulated. In this study, the only vessel completely isolated before sealing was the splenic artery. Three overlapping seals were applied to this vessel. A more recent study supported the adequacy of a single seal on the carotid artery.[48] Therefore, judgment should be exercised to the proximity of other vital structures and manufacturer's recommendations on vessel size. Similar results supporting the efficacy of vessels sealing devices have been seen with partial liver lobectomies, partial lung lobectomies, uterine horns and bodies, ovarian pedicles and pancreas.[22,45,50,52-54]

SUMMARY

- When understood and used properly, stapling and vessel sealing devices can increase confidence of the surgeon, precision, decrease surgical time, and contribute positively to the outcome of the surgery, especially in the critically ill patient.
- The use of surgical stapling and vessel sealing devices should not replace good surgical and soft tissue handling techniques.

- It is the responsibility of the surgical team and the surgeon to possess the prerequisite knowledge for the use of stapling and vessel sealing instruments and to be aware of the limitations and indications of each of these individual devices.

REFERENCES

1. Schwartz A. Historical and veterinary perspectives of surgical stapling. Vet Clin North Am Small Anim Pract 1994;24:225–46.
2. Schwarz A. Mechanical staplers: alternative to conventional sutures? DVM Magazine 1982;13:30.
3. Lipscomb V. Surgical staplers: toy or tool? Practice 2012;34:472–9.
4. Pavletic MM, Schwarz A. Stapling instruments. Vet Clin North Am Small Anim Pract 1994;24:247–78.
5. Tobias KM. Surgical stapling devices in veterinary medicine: a review. Vet Surg 2007;36:341–9.
6. Pavletic MM. Surgical stapling devices in small animal surgery. Compend Contin Educ Small Anim Pract 1990;12:1724–41.
7. Ullman SL, Pavletic MM, Clark GN. Open intestinal anastomosis with surgical stapling equipment in 24 dogs and cats. Vet Surg 1991;20:385–91.
8. Lewis DD, Ellison GW, Bellah JR. Partial hepatectomy using stapling instruments. J Am Anim Hosp Assoc 1987;23:597–602.
9. LaRue SM, Withrow SJ, Wykes PM. Lung resection using surgical staples in dogs and cats. Vet Surg 1987;16:238–40.
10. Clark GN. Gastric surgery with surgical stapling instruments. Vet Clin North Am Small Anim Pract 1994;24:279–304.
11. Ullman SL. Surgical stapling of the small intestine. Vet Clin North Am Small Anim Pract 1994;24:305–22.
12. Walshaw R. Stapling techniques in pulmonary surgery. Vet Clin North Am Small Anim Pract 1994;24:334–66.
13. Monnet E, Orton EC. Surgical stapling devices in cardiovascular surgery. Vet Clin North Am Small Anim Pract 1994;24:367–74.
14. Bellah JR. Surgical stapling of the spleen, pancreas, liver and urogenital tract. Vet Clin North Am Small Anim Pract 1994;24:375–94.
15. Pavletic MM. Stapling in esophageal surgery. Vet Clin North Am Small Anim Pract 1994;24:395–412.
16. Kudisch M, Pavletic MM. Subtotal colectomy with surgical stapling instruments via a trans-cecal approach for treatment of acquired megacolon in cats. Vet Surg 1993;22:457–63.
17. Kudisch M. Surgical stapling of large intestines. Vet Clin North Am Small Anim Pract 1994;24:323–34.
18. Fucci V, Newton JC, Hedlund CS, et al. Rectal surgery in the cat – comparison of suture versus staple technique through a dorsal approach. J Am Anim Hosp Assoc 1992;28:519–26.
19. Schmiedt CW. Suture material, tissue staplers, ligation devices, and closure methods. In: Tobias KM, Johnston SA, editors. Veterinary surgery: small animal, vol. 1, 1st edition. Philadelphia: WB Saunders; 2012. p. 196–200.
20. Swiderski J, Withrow S. A novel surgical stapling technique for rectal mass removal: a retrospective analysis. J Am Anim Hosp Assoc 1999;45:67–71.
21. Covey JL, Degner DA, Jackson AH, et al. Hilar liver resection in dogs. Vet Surg 2009;38:104–11.

22. Risellada M, Ellison GW, Bacon NJ, et al. Comparison of 5 surgical techniques for partial liver lobectomy in the dog for intraoperative blood loss and surgical time. Vet Surg 2010;39:856–62.

23. Mayhew PD, Weisse C. Liver and biliary system. In: Tobias KM, Johnston SA, editors. Veterinary surgery: small animal, vol. 2, 1st edition. Philadelphia: WB Saunders; 2012. p. 1601–23.

24. Pavia PR, Koval-McClaran J, Lamb K. Outcome following liver lobectomy using thoracoabdominal staplers in cats. J Small Anim Pract 2014;55:22–7.

25. Eisele J, McClaran JK, Runge JJ, et al. Evaluation of risk factors for morbidity and mortality after pylorectomy and gastroduodenostomy in dogs. Vet Surg 2010;39:261–7.

26. Belandria GA, Pavletic MM, Boulay JP, et al. Gastropexy with an automatic stapling instrument for the treatment of gastric dilatation volvulus in 20 dogs. Can Vet J 2009;50:733–40.

27. Ployart S, Libermann S, Doran I, et al. Thoracoscopic resection of right auricular masses in dogs: 9 cases (2003–2011). J Am Vet Med Assoc 2013;242:237–41.

28. Jardel N, Hidalgo A, Leperlier D, et al. One stage functional end-to-end stapled intestinal anastomosis and resection performed by nonexpert surgeons for the treatment of small intestinal obstruction in 30 dogs. Vet Surg 2011;40:216–22.

29. White RN. Modified functional end-to-end stapled intestinal anastomosis: technique and clinical response in 15 dogs. J Small Anim Pract 2008;49:274–81.

30. Hess JL. Use of a simultaneous ligating-dividing-stapling instrument for ovariohysterectomy. Vet Med Small Anim Clin 1979;74:1480.

31. Hess JL, DeYoung DW, Grier RL. Use of mechanical staples in veterinary thoracic surgery. J Am Anim Hosp Assoc 1979;15:539–73.

32. Toombs JP, Clark KM. Basic operative techniques. In: Slatter D, editor. Textbook of small animal surgery, vol. 1, 3rd edition. Philadelphia: WB Saunders; 2003. p. 199.

33. Borenstein N, Behr L, Chetboul V, et al. Minimally invasive patent ductus arteriosus occlusion in 5 dogs. Vet Surg 2004;33:309–13.

34. Corti LB, Merkley D, Nelson OL, et al. Retrospective evaluation of occlusion of patent ductus arteriosus with Hemoclips in 20 dogs. J Am Anim Hosp Assoc 2000;36:548–55.

35. Waldron DR. Skin and fascia staple closure. Vet Clin North Am Small Anim Pract 1994;24:413–24.

36. Frey TN, Hoelzler MG, Scavelli TD, et al. Risk factors for surgical site infection-inflammation in dogs undergoing surgery for rupture of the cranial cruciate ligament: 902 cases (2005–2006). J Am Vet Med Assoc 2010;236:88–94.

37. Torfs S, Levet T, Delesalle C, et al. Risk factors for incisional complications after exploratory celiotomy in horses: do skin staples increase the risk? Vet Surg 2010;39:616–20.

38. Coolman BR, Ehrhart N, Marretta SM. Use of skin staples for rapid closure of gastrointestinal incisions in the treatment of canine linear foreign bodies. J Am Anim Hosp Assoc 2000;36:542–7.

39. Coolman BR, Ehrhart N, Pijanowski GJ, et al. Comparison of skin staples with sutures for anastomosis of the small intestine in dogs. Vet Surg 2000;29:293–302.

40. Coolman BR, Maretta SM, Pijanowski GJ, et al. Evaluation of a skin stapler for belt-loop gastropexy in dogs. J Am Anim Hosp Assoc 1999;35:440–4.

41. Mayhew PD. Recent advances in soft tissue minimally invasive surgery. J Small Anim Pract 2014;55:75–83.

42. Landsdowne JL, Monnet E, Twedt DC, et al. Thoracoscopic lung lobectomy for treatment of lung tumors in dogs. Vet Surg 2005;34:530–5.

43. Crumbaker DM, Rooney MB, Case JB. Thoracoscopic subtotal pericardectomy and right atrial mass resection in a dog. J Am Vet Med Assoc 2010;237:551–4.
44. Rivier P, Monnet E. Use of a vessel sealant device for splenectomy in dogs. Vet Surg 2010;40:102–5.
45. Mayhew PD, Culp WT, Pascoe PJ, et al. Use of the Ligasure vessel-sealing device for thoracoscopic peripheral lung biopsy in healthy dogs. Vet Surg 2012;41: 523–8.
46. Sackman JE. Surgical modalities: laser, radiofrequency, ultrasonic and electro-surgery. In: Tobias KM, Johnston SA, editors. Veterinary surgery: small animal, vol. 1, 1st edition. Philadelphia: WB Saunders; 2012. p. 183.
47. Landman J, Kerbl K, Rehman J, et al. Evaluation of a vessel sealing system, bi-polar electrosurgery, Harmonic Scalpel, titanium clips, endoscopic gastro-intestinal anastomosis vascular staples and sutures for arterial and venous ligation in a porcine model. J Urol 2003;169:697–700.
48. Matz BM, Tillson DM, Boothe HW, et al. Effect of vascular seal configuration using the LigaSure on arterial challenge pressure, time for seal creation, and histologic features. Vet Surg 2014;43:761–4.
49. Ohlund M, Hoglund O, Olsson U, et al. Laparoscopic ovariectomy in dogs: a comparison of the LigaSure and the Sonosurg systems. J Small Anim Pract 2011;52:290–4.
50. Wouters EG, Buishand FO, Kik M, et al. Use of a bipolar vessel-sealing device in resection of canine insulinoma. J Small Anim Pract 2011;52:139–45.
51. Silverman EM, Read RW, Boyle CR, et al. Histologic comparison of canine skin biopsies collected during monopolar electrosurgery, CO2 laser, radiowave radio-surgery, skin biopsy punch and scalpel. Vet Surg 2007;36:50–6.
52. Monarski CJ, Jaffe MH, Kass PH. Decreased surgical time with a vessel sealing device versus a surgical stapler in performance of canine splenectomy. J Am Anim Hosp Assoc 2014;50:42–5.
53. Barrera JS, Monnet E. Effectiveness of a bipolar vessel sealant device for sealing uterine horns and bodies from dogs. Am J Vet Res 2012;73:302–5.
54. Coisman JG, Case JB, Shih A, et al. Comparison of surgical variable in cats under-going single-incision laparoscopic ovariectomy using a LigaSure or extracorporeal suture versus open ovariectomy. Vet Surg 2014;43:38–44.

Current Concepts in Hepatobiliary Surgery

Harry W. Boothe Jr, DVM, MS

KEYWORDS

- Hepatobiliary surgery • Hepatic mass lesions • Liver biopsy • Partial hepatectomy
- Cholecystectomy • Cholecystoenterostomy • Choledochotomy

KEY POINTS

- Knowledge of the anatomy of the liver and biliary tract helps minimize complications associated with hepatobiliary surgery.
- Information important for planning partial hepatectomies to treat hepatic masses includes distribution of mass lesions; histologic diagnosis; and patient oncotic, blood typing/cross-matching, and coagulation status.
- Goals of extrahepatic biliary surgery include confirmation of the underlying disease process (eg, biliary mucocele, cholecystitis, and bile duct obstruction; trauma; or leakage) establishment of a patent biliary system, and minimization of perioperative complications.
- Veterinary patients undergoing either extensive liver resection or correction of biliary tract obstruction or leakage tend to have an extensive list of risk factors associated with the primary condition and the surgical procedure.

INTRODUCTION AND ANATOMIC CONSIDERATIONS

Hepatobiliary surgery in dogs and cats may be used to investigate or treat various conditions of the liver and biliary tract including persistent hepatic disease, hepatic abscessation, hepatic mass lesions, gallbladder mucocele, cholecystitis, biliary leakage, and extrahepatic biliary obstruction. Surgical procedures performed include hepatic biopsy, partial hepatectomy, cholecystotomy, cholecystectomy, cholecystoenterostomy, and choledochotomy. Although liver transplantation is not currently performed clinically in dogs and cats, information gleaned from its use in research dogs has provided valuable information to the clinical veterinary surgeon.[1] Knowledge of the anatomy of the liver and biliary tract helps minimize complications associated with hepatobiliary surgery.

The author has nothing to disclose.
Wilford and Kate Bailey Small Animal Teaching Hospital, Department of Clinical Sciences, College of Veterinary Medicine, 1220 Wire Road, Auburn, AL 36849-5540, USA
E-mail address: boothhw@auburn.edu

Vet Clin Small Anim 45 (2015) 463–475
http://dx.doi.org/10.1016/j.cvsm.2015.01.001   vetsmall.theclinics.com

The liver is the largest gland in the body and has exocrine (bile) and endocrine function. It is divided into four lobes (left, right, quadrate, and caudate), four sublobes, and two processes by deep fissures. The left hepatic lobe, comprised of the left lateral and medial sublobes, which may be joined by a bridge of liver tissue dorsally, forms nearly one-half of the total liver mass. The right hepatic lobe is smaller than the left and has the right lateral and medial sublobes. The right lateral lobe is often fused to the right medial lobe and the caudate process of the caudate lobe. The right medial lobe is variably fused to the quadrate lobe. The quadrate lobe lies almost on the midline, and its lateral aspect forms one side of the gallbladder fossa. The caudate lobe is composed of the caudate and papillary processes and the connecting isthmus. The isthmus is located between the dorsally located caudal vena cava and the more ventral portal vein. The caudate process forms the most caudal portion of the liver, whereas the papillary process lies in the lesser curvature of the stomach.[2] From a surgical perspective, the liver may be grouped into three subdivisions: left (left lateral and medial lobes) comprising approximately 44% of liver volume, central (quadrate and right medial lobes), and right (right lateral and caudate lobes), each comprising about 28% of liver volume.

The portal vein provides the functional blood supply to the liver. It divides into left and right branches in the dog, with the left branch supplying the central and left divisions. The feline portal vein divides into right, left, and central branches. The hepatic artery provides nutritional supply to hepatic parenchyma and bile ducts.[1] Each canine sublobe is supplied by a single hepatic artery and at least one lobar portal vein.[3]

The biliary system begins at the hepatic canaliculi, with up to eight hepatic ducts, although three or four hepatic ducts was more commonly observed, joining to form the bile duct.[4] The initial hepatic duct to enter the bile duct usually is the right medial hepatic duct.[4] The gallbladder is connected to the bile duct via the cystic duct, which tends to be greater than 5 mm long in most dogs.[4] After passing intramurally within the duodenum for approximately 2 cm, the bile duct opens approximately 3 to 6 cm aborad to the pylorus.

LIVER BIOPSY CONSIDERATIONS
Indications and Contraindications

Diagnosis of most liver diseases requires histopathologic examination of liver tissue.[5] Diffuse liver diseases may be sampled randomly, but focal lesions require careful selective sampling.[5] Ideally, the patient's coagulation status should be assessed before a liver biopsy is performed.[5] Significant bleeding complications have been observed in dogs and cats with thrombocytopenia (platelets $<80 \times 10^3/\mu L$) undergoing ultrasound-guided liver biopsies.[6] The liver may be evaluated via fine-needle aspiration (cytology) or biopsy (histopathology). Ultrasound-guided fine-needle aspirations for cytologic examination of the liver have been shown to have serious limitations when used to identify the primary disease process in dogs and cats with clinical evidence of liver disease.[7] Hepatic cytologic samples are more reliable for diffuse hepatic disease, especially neoplasia, and less reliable for inflammation, necrosis, and hyperplasia.[8]

Technique

Liver biopsies are performed frequently and use various techniques in dogs and cats, including needle core, laparoscopic, and surgical biopsy. An ideal liver biopsy should be of proper size and taken from a location that represents the primary liver pathology.[5] Samples from multiple lobes are often preferred. In addition to tissues for histopathology, samples may also be obtained for microbiologic testing or quantification of copper or other metals.[5,9] Comparison of needle and wedge hepatic biopsy techniques has been made.[10] Ultrasound-guided percutaneous techniques using a needle core biopsy are one option for sampling the liver. Findings in needle biopsy samples taken with ultrasound guidance or at laparotomy concurred with the definitive diagnosis in 48% of dogs and cats in an earlier study.[10]

Laparoscopic liver biopsies may be obtained from grossly abnormal areas of the liver, particularly near the periphery of the liver lobes. Advantages of laparoscopic biopsy over laparotomy sampling include lower patient morbidity and decreased infection rate, postoperative pain, and hospitalization time.[5,11]

Surgical methods of sampling the liver include ligature (suture) fracture or guillotine technique and biopsy punch technique. Surgical liver biopsies should be taken early during the laparotomy to minimize hepatocellular changes from prolonged anesthesia or manipulation of intestine.[12] Advantages of surgical biopsy techniques include enhanced exposure and ability to manipulate tissues, obtain large sample sizes, and monitor biopsy sites for bleeding.[5] Hepatic biopsies obtained via laparotomy are the largest of any of the methods described and should provide adequate tissue for various analyses.[5,9]

The ligature (suture) fracture or guillotine technique is performed on the periphery of a liver lobe, with variably sized samples obtained (**Fig. 1**). Use of a pretied ligating loop to obtain liver biopsies was found to be versatile and safe in dogs.[13] The biopsy punch technique results in collection of partial-thickness samples (ie, less than half the thickness of the lobe) of liver, usually from its ventral surface.[3] Lesions located away from the periphery of the liver may be sampled using the biopsy punch. Hemostasis is provided by suture (ligature fracture technique), omental coverage of the biopsy site (either surgical biopsy technique), electrocoagulation (either technique), or gelatin sponge (either technique).

Complications

Hemorrhage is the most frequently described complication, although abscessation of an hepatic biopsy site has been reported and observed by the author.[14]

HEPATIC ABSCESSATION

Hepatic abscessation in dogs or cats is reported relatively uncommonly, with middle-aged to older dogs and cats usually being described.[3,14,15] Abdominal ultrasonography is a relatively sensitive tool for diagnosis. Solitary hepatic abscessation may

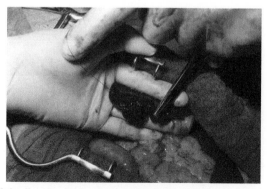

Fig. 1. A biopsy of the liver is obtained using the ligature fracture (guillotine) method. The isolated portion of liver distal to the suture material (2-0 PDS) is excised using scissors.

be more common in dogs than in cats.[14] Microbiologic sampling often yields variable isolates, although *Escherichia coli* is frequently found.

Technique

Diagnostic and treatment principles include complete evaluation to determine any concurrent disease process (eg, neoplasia) and the extent and number of abscesses, use of appropriate broad-spectrum antimicrobials, and possibly surgery. Surgical intervention involves partial hepatectomy or drainage procedures (eg, omentalization). Hepatic abscessation in dogs does not seem to have an anatomic site predilection or to be associated with neoplasia, whereas cats have their right hepatic lobes more commonly affected. Multiple abscess sites and concurrent hepatobiliary neoplasia are more likely in cats.[15]

HEPATIC MASS LESIONS

Primary hepatic neoplasia is reported to occur in 0.6% to 2.6% of dogs and 1.5% to 2.3% of cats, with biliary neoplasia seen less frequently.[3] Four general types of primary hepatobiliary neoplasia are described: (1) hepatocellular, (2) cholangiocellular, (3) neuroendocrine, and (4) mesenchymal. Primary hepatic neoplasms in dogs can be classified and differentiated using immunohistochemical stains as markers representative of hepatocytic and cholangiocytic lineages.[16] Metastatic tumors of the liver are more common than primary tumors, with approximately 30% of dogs having hepatic metastatic tumors. The presence of hepatic masses may be noted on abdominal ultrasonography, although advanced imaging (eg, computed tomography or MRI) provides information to help discern tumor location, distribution, and potentially differentiate malignant from benign masses.[3] Determination of specific tissue types is facilitated by fine-needle aspiration of cells or needle core, laparoscopic, or surgical biopsy. Reported rates for correct diagnoses of hepatic masses range from up to 50% for fine-needle aspiration to 70% for needle core samples.[3]

Hepatocellular Tumors

Hepatocellular tumors are the most common primary hepatic tumor of dogs, representing 50% to 70% of all nonhematopoietic neoplasms (**Fig. 2**). Three forms of hepatocellular tumors are described: (1) massive (61%), (2) nodular (29%), and (3) diffuse (10%). Metastasis is more common with nodular or diffuse forms (93%) than with the massive form (36%). Anatomic distribution of lesions with the massive form is

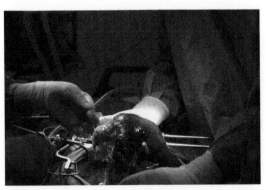

Fig. 2. Omental adhesions are dissected from this massive hepatocellular carcinoma present in the left lateral lobe of a 12-year-old Labrador retriever.

approximately 67% in left lobes, 15% in central lobes, and 18% in right lobes. Hepatocellular tumors with hepatic progenitor cellular characteristics tend to be poorly differentiated and aggressive in behavior.[16] Hepatocellular tumors are reported less commonly in cats, representing less than 25% of primary hepatic neoplasms. Hepatocellular adenomas are more common than carcinomas in cats, whereas hepatocellular carcinomas in dogs are seen twice as frequently as are hepatocellular adenomas.

Surgical resection is the preferred treatment of massive hepatocellular carcinoma in dogs, generally carrying a favorable prognosis.[3] Because of likely incomplete surgical resection and high metastatic rate, surgery is not a good option for nodular or diffuse forms of hepatocellular carcinoma in dogs.[3] Surgical challenges presented by central or right-sided masses are usually greater than those presented by left-sided masses.

Cholangiocellular (Bile Duct) Tumors

Cholangiocellular tumors account for approximately 30% of primary hepatic tumors in dogs. Cholangiocellular carcinomas are thought to be derived from differentiated mucin-producing cholangiocytes, normally present in larger bile ducts. Bile duct tumors tend to exhibit infiltrative growth, vascular invasion, and intrahepatic or distant metastasis.[16] Most canine cholangiocellular carcinomas are intrahepatic in location. Massive and nodular types occur with relative similar frequency, with diffuse types being less common. Bile duct tumors are the most common primary hepatic neoplasm in cats, with the benign adenoma, biliary cystadenoma, being about twice as common as cholangiocellular carcinomas (**Fig. 3**).[3] Benign bile duct tumors in cats have a better prognosis than malignant forms.

Neuroendocrine Tumors

Neuroendocrine tumors account for approximately 15% of canine and 4% of feline primary hepatic tumors.[3] They are thought to be derived from pre-existing neuroendocrine cells in the biliary epithelium.[16] Neuroendocrine carcinomas are aggressive tumors and are associated with a poor prognosis.[3] Diffuse liver involvement and peritoneal carcinomatosis are frequent features of canine neuroendocrine carcinoma. More feline neuroendocrine carcinomas are extrahepatic in location, with involvement of the bile ducts or gallbladder being observed.[3]

Mesenchymal Tumors

A variety of mesenchymal tumors of the liver in dogs and cats have been described. They account for approximately 10% of primary hepatic neoplasms in dogs and cats.[3] Primary hepatic hemangiosarcoma may be seen in dogs and cats, but less

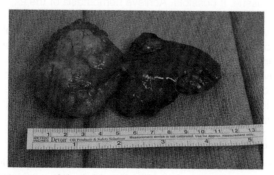

Fig. 3. Partial hepatectomy of the left medial lobe in an 18-year-old domestic shorthair cat (DSH) revealed biliary cystadenomas.

commonly than the metastatic form from spleen or other organs.[3] Other primary hepatic mesenchymal tumors include leiomyosarcoma, osteosarcoma, and fibrosarcoma.

PERIOPERATIVE CONSIDERATIONS FOR PARTIAL HEPATECTOMY

Although research dogs have been shown to tolerate extended hepatectomy, with up to 90% of the hepatic mass being excised, partial hepatectomy in clinical patients usually involves removal of one or two hepatic lobes.[17] Information important for planning partial or complete hepatic lobectomies includes distribution of mass lesions; histologic diagnosis; and patient oncotic, blood typing/cross-matching, and coagulation status. Using a team approach to provide patient care in the perioperative period seemingly has beneficial effects. The team usually consists of two experienced surgeons and one anesthetist. Planning by the team should include having appropriate fluid and blood products available, proper patient instrumentation for anesthetic monitoring, presurgical calculation of the trigger point of blood loss for administration of blood products, having special surgical equipment available, and an immediate postoperative patient management strategy. Having specific information about location of the mass (ie, left, right, or central) helps make presurgical planning more accurate and appropriate.

Indications

Partial hepatectomy is performed for smaller, more peripherally located lesions. Complete hepatic lobectomy is technically easier to perform on the left hepatic lobes, because of their more accessible hilus.

Technique

Adequate exposure is essential to success of hepatic lobectomy surgery. Extension of the ventral midline abdominal approach through or along the xiphoid process and through the ventral diaphragm into the thoracic cavity or paracostally on the affected side may improve access to the affected hepatic lobe. Assess extent of adhesions to surrounding tissues and proximity of the mass to the hilus. Transect ligamentous attachments to the affected lobe. Ligate branches of the portal and hepatic veins and hepatic artery and hepatic ducts to the affected hepatic lobes. When central lobes are affected, confirm the location of the portal vein branches to the right and left divisions, because these branches need to be preserved. Confirm the proximity of the caudal vena cava and bile duct to the affected lobes. Initiate parenchymal dissection, using fingers or suction tip as close to the hilus as required to achieve a grossly normal margin of hepatic tissue, if possible. Achieve hemostasis of the exposed hepatic parenchyma before final transection of the mass, because traction on the affected lobe enhances visibility of the excision site. No significant bleeding should be noted from the cut surface of the liver after partial or complete hepatic lobectomy.[3] Confirm patency of the bile duct and portal venous and hepatic arterial branches to remaining hepatic lobes. Lavage the peritoneal cavity with warm saline before closure to remove dislodged blood clots. Postoperative management should include appropriate analgesic administration, attention to blood volume and oncotic status, and conscientious antimicrobial therapy.

Complications and Management

Possible complications of partial or complete hepatic lobectomy include hemorrhage and trauma, including occlusion, of the biliary tract or portal vasculature to the remaining liver. Hemorrhage is a common and occasionally life-threatening complication of hepatic surgery.[18] Hepatic vascular anatomy presents challenges in hemostasis.[18] Most of the blood flow to the liver is via large, thin-walled branches of the portal vein. Additionally the right liver lobes are adhered to a lengthy section of the caudal vena cava.[18] Dissection around the caudal vena cava or portal branches may result in brisk hemorrhage. Fracture or incision of hepatic tissue causes parenchymal bleeding that is challenging to control, even with stapling or vessel sealing equipment.[18] Options for achieving hemostasis include one or more of the following: direct pressure; use of topical hemostatic agents; hemostatic clips; ligations; stapling equipment (eg, thoracoabdominal stapler with vascular cartridge); and electrosurgical devices, including vessel sealing systems.

Direct pressure is the simplest technique to address parenchymal hemorrhage during liver surgery.[18] Pressure with a moistened laparotomy sponge can be applied to the traumatized liver surface for several minutes. Slowly remove the sponge to avoid clot disturbance.[18] Various topical hemostatic agents (eg, gelatin sponge, oxidized regenerated cellulose) can help achieve hemorrhage control from the hepatic parenchyma. Hemostatic clips are more easily placed than ligatures, because they require less dissection and are easier to place in deep, confined locations.[18] Proper selection of clip size and good application technique are essential to avoid clip dislodgement.[18] Length of the compressed clip should be two to three times the diameter of the vessel.[18] Direct vascular ligation placement (eg, on the lobar portal and hepatic veins and hepatic artery) is more versatile and effective than is an encircling ligature around the base of the liver. Encircling ligatures are only recommended for use in small dogs and cats and for removal of left hepatic lobes.[18]

Use of stapling equipment is usually an efficient process, although challenges associated with its use in partial hepatectomy surgery include limited accessibility of the area to be stapled and dimensions (width and thickness) of the hepatic tissue to be divided. Stapler use does not require blunt dissection of hepatic tissue or isolation of specific lobar vessels and hepatic ducts.[18] A variety of electrosurgical units may be used during partial hepatectomies. Bipolar or monopolar handpieces may have applicability to hepatic lobectomies. Vessel sealing systems (eg, LigaSure [Covidien, Minneapolis, MN]) are effective on arteries up to 5-mm diameter and veins up to 7-mm diameter.[18] Collagen and elastin are effectively melted, creating a permanent seal after a single application.[18] Other vessel sealing technologies used in hepatic surgery include an ultrasound-activated scalpel or LASER [Aesculight, LLC, Woodinville, WA] energy systems.

EXTRAHEPATIC BILIARY SURGERY AND POTENTIAL COMPLICATIONS

Goals of extrahepatic biliary surgery include confirmation of the underlying disease process (eg, biliary mucocele, cholecystitis, and bile duct obstruction, trauma, or leakage), establishment of a patent biliary system, and minimization of perioperative complications.[18] Confirming the extent (partial vs complete) and the cause of biliary obstruction in dogs and cats is challenging and frequently involves multiple diagnostic modalities. Although information gained from serum biochemical testing results and abdominal ultrasonography is helpful in assessing the extrahepatic biliary tract, hepatobiliary scintigraphy may be needed to differentiate biliary obstruction from hepatocellular disease or damage and determine whether biliary tract dilation indicates a resolved or ongoing obstruction.[19,20] Fashioning a rational plan to treat biliary obstruction is best accomplished by knowing the cause, extent, and likely duration of the obstruction (**Fig. 4**). Information from experimental dogs suggests that delaying primary surgical repair of an obstructed bile duct for at least 10 days after onset of obstruction may be appropriate because of wound healing considerations.[21]

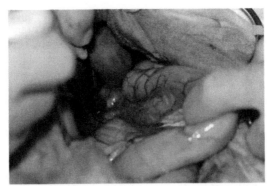

Fig. 4. This dilated biliary tract was observed in a 5-month-old Boxer with biliary obstruction caused by intestinal pythiosis.

Leakage from the biliary tract results in bile peritonitis. Bile salts are toxic to tissue, resulting in permeability changes and necrosis.[19] Although nonseptic bile peritonitis has a milder clinical course than septic bile peritonitis, timely exploration and correction of the source of bile leakage is indicated.[19] Successful primary repair of ruptured bile ducts has been reported in dogs.[22] However, treatment of bile duct leakage may be more predictably managed with biliary rerouting and ligation of the bile duct because of the technical challenges and complications of primary repair.[19] Surgical options relating to the extrahepatic biliary tract include cholecystectomy; cholecystotomy; biliary rerouting procedures, including cholecystoenterostomy (cholecystoduodenostomy or cholecystojejunostomy) and choledochoduodenostomy; and use of tube or stents in the gallbladder (cholecystostomy tube) or bile duct (choledochal stents).

The gallbladder wall does not seal well immediately after cholecystocentesis or cholecystotomy, and repair of hepatic, cystic, or bile ducts is technically demanding and characterized by a high rate of failure, in part because of ischemic damage to the bile duct.[19,23] Tubes or stents in the extrahepatic biliary tract usually are placed surgically, rather than endoscopically, in dogs and cats.

Potential complications of extrahepatic biliary surgery include hemorrhage, dehiscence and leakage (bile peritonitis), obstruction of the bile duct, stricture of the biliary enteric anastomotic stoma, ascending cholangiohepatitis, recurrent cholelithiasis, and altered gastrointestinal physiology.[19,24]

Cholecystectomy

Indications
The most common surgical procedure performed on the gallbladder of dogs and cats is cholecystectomy. The most common indication for cholecystectomy in the dog is biliary mucocele (**Fig. 5**). The primary indication for feline cholecystectomy is necrotizing cholecystitis, although cholecystectomy for cholelithiasis has been reported (**Fig. 6**).[25]

Technique
The relative difficulty associated with cholecystectomy in dogs and cats pertains, in part, to the extent of adhesion formation between the gallbladder and surrounding tissues (eg, liver, greater omentum, falciform ligament) and the status, including integrity, of the gallbladder (**Fig. 7**). Cholecystectomy is usually performed via laparotomy in dogs and cats, although a laparoscopic procedure has been described in dogs.[26]

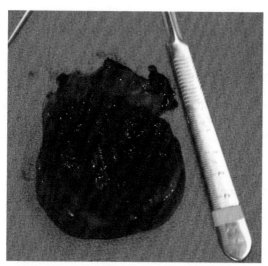

Fig. 5. A gallbladder from a 3-year-old Shetland Sheepdog with a biliary mucocele has been incised to reveal its contents.

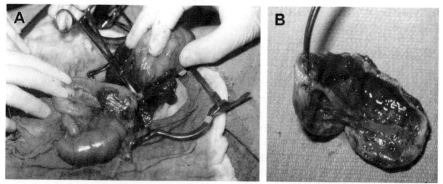

Fig. 6. (A) Cholecystectomy is being performed in a 13-year-old DSH with necrotizing chole-cystitis. Note evidence of adhesion formation between the gallbladder and proximal duo-denum. (B) The diseased gallbladder has been incised to reveal its mucosal surface.

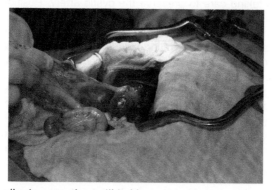

Fig. 7. Omental adhesions to the gallbladder are evident in this 3-year-old Shetland Sheepdog with a biliary mucocele.

Dissect the gallbladder from the hepatic fossa using blunt and sharp dissection. Achieve hemorrhage control of the hepatic fossa via local pressure, electrosurgery, and topical hemostatic agents. Ensure patency of the bile duct by passing a catheter (eg, 5F red rubber catheter) through the bile duct in a normograde (preferred technique) or retrograde fashion. Retrograde catheter passage requires a duodenotomy to access the duodenal papilla. Dissection to the level of the cystic duct usually reveals the cystic artery, which is ligated or occluded collectively with the cystic duct with an appropriately sized vascular clip. Confirm hemostasis and perform intraperitoneal lavage before closure.

Cholecystotomy

Indications
Cholecystotomy occasionally may be performed to obtain full-thickness biopsies or mucosal cultures of the gallbladder, explore the gallbladder or cystic duct, remove choleliths or sludge in an otherwise normal gallbladder, or normograde flush the bile duct.[19]

Technique
Pack off the gallbladder and incise it at its apex. Evacuate contents and flush the gallbladder and cystic and bile ducts. Retrograde flushing of the bile duct via the duodenal papilla helps ensure evacuation of the entire biliary tract. Close the incision with a simple continuous pattern using synthetic monofilament absorbable suture material.[3] Cover the incision with greater omentum.

Cholecystoenterostomy/Choledochoduodenostomy

Indications
Surgical treatment of extrahepatic biliary obstruction or leakage may include cholecystoenterostomy. Creating a connection between the lumen of the gallbladder and either the duodenum or jejunum is achieved. Although reconstruction of the bile duct has been successfully performed experimentally in dogs using various materials, treatment of a clinical patient with bile duct obstruction or leakage often includes a biliary enteric anastomotic procedure in concert with ligation of the bile duct.[27,28] Alternatively, primary bile duct repair or choledochotomy are potential options.

Technique
Cholecystoduodenostomy is generally accepted as the most physiologic technique to achieve biliary enteric anastomoses in dogs and cats.[29] Dissect the gallbladder from the hepatic fossa taking care to preserve the cystic artery. Position the gallbladder adjacent to the antimesenteric aspect of the duodenum without obstructing the cystic duct, and create matching incisions in the wall of the gallbladder and the duodenum. Appose mucosal surfaces of the gallbladder and duodenum using a simple continuous pattern of 4-0 synthetic absorbable suture material or a surgical stapling device to create the stoma. Stoma size should be greater than or equal to 2.5 cm in length to prevent stricturing and minimize ascending cholangiohepatitis. If tension is noted during attempted mobilization of the gallbladder, a cholecystojejunostomy may be the preferred technique. If the bile duct has dilated because of partial or complete obstruction at its duodenal termination, choledochoduodenostomy or reanastomosis of the bile duct to an unaffected portion of the duodenum may be an option.[30]

Choledochotomy/Choledochal or Cholecystostomy Tubes

Choledochotomy and placement of choledochal tubes has been reported in dogs and cats.[22,31,32] Closure of the choledochotomy is achieved over a red rubber catheter of appropriate diameter (usually 5–8F catheter) using either synthetic monofilament absorbable or nonabsorbable suture material. Suture used is often 3-0 or 4-0 in size, with a simple interrupted or continuous pattern. Suturing the tube to the duodenal wall may extend the duration of stenting. Removal of the stent may be achieved endoscopically.

Indications

Obstructive cholangiolithiasis or pancreatitis is the usual inciting reason for placement of choledochal tubes. Cholecystostomy tubes provide temporary diversion of bile from the gallbladder to a closed collection system.[3] Such tubes are considered only when the gallbladder wall is deemed to be healthy.[3]

Technique

Tube placement may be accomplished via laparotomy or laparoscopic-assisted. Insert a pigtail or Foley catheter into the apex of the gallbladder and place a purse-string suture around the base of the catheter to minimize leakage. Exit the abdomen just caudal to the costal arch, and secure the tube to the skin using a friction suture. Attach the tube to a sterile collection system.

OUTCOMES FOR PATIENTS UNDERGOING HEPATOBILIARY SURGERY

Information regarding outcome is available for selected hepatobiliary surgical procedures.[3,14,15,18,19,25,29,31–34] Veterinary patients undergoing either extensive liver resection or correction of biliary tract obstruction or leakage tend to have an extensive list of risk factors associated with the primary condition and the surgical procedure. Anesthetic management of the dog or cat with hepatobiliary dysfunction tends to be challenging, in part because hepatic disease impacts many body functions. Dogs undergoing cholecystectomy were not shown to have any greater number of anesthesia complications than were dogs that underwent other hepatic surgeries.[35] Dogs or cats with hepatic mass lesions have oncologic and perioperative factors that influence prognosis.

SUMMARY

Surgery of the liver and extrahepatic biliary tract presents technical challenges to the veterinary clinician. Such challenges include gaining access to the lesion; dealing with highly vascular, friable hepatic tissue; potentially difficult-to-heal tissue (eg, extrahepatic biliary tract); and the impact of the primary condition on the patient's response to surgery. Enhancement of outcome and minimizing potential complications can be achieved by performing accurate preoperative patient assessment and treatment, using a team approach to the surgery and perioperative care, demonstrating flexibility to change intraoperative plans, and following a comprehensive postoperative management plan.

REFERENCES

1. Lu HW, Chen YB, Li YM, et al. Role of hepatic arterial ischaemia in biliary fibrosis following liver transplantation. Chin Med J 2010;123(7):907–11.
2. Evans HE, deLahunta A. The digestive apparatus and abdomen. In: Evans HE, Alexander de Lahunta, editors. Miller's anatomy of the dog. 4th edition. St Louis (MO): Saunders, an imprint of Elsevier; 2013. p. 327–33.

3. Mayhew PD, Weisse C. Liver and biliary system. In: Tobias KM, Johnston SA, editors. Veterinary surgery: small animal. St Louis (MO): Saunders, an imprint of Elsevier; 2012. p. 1601–23.

4. Imagawa T, Ueno T, Tsuka T, et al. Anatomical variations of the extrahepatic ducts in dogs: knowledge for surgical procedures. J Vet Med Sci 2001;72(3):339–41.

5. Rothuizen J, Twedt DC. Liver biopsy techniques. Vet Clin North Am Small Anim Pract 2009;39:469–80.

6. Bigge LA, Brown DJ, Penninck DG. Correlation between coagulation profile findings and bleeding complications after ultrasound-guided biopsies: 434 Cases (1993-1996). J Am Anim Hosp Assoc 2001;37:228–33.

7. Wang KY, Panciera DL, Al-Rukibat RK, et al. Accuracy of ultrasound-guided fine-needle aspiration of the liver and cytologic findings in dogs and cats: 97 cases (1990-2000). J Am Vet Med Assoc 2004;224:75–8.

8. Bahr KL, Sharkey LC, Murakami T, et al. Accuracy of US-guided FNA of focal liver lesions in dogs: 140 cases (2005-2008). J Am Anim Hosp Assoc 2013;49:190–6.

9. Johnston AN, Center SA, McDonough SP. Influence of biopsy specimen size, tissue fixation, and assay variation on copper, iron, and zinc concentrations in canine livers. Am J Vet Res 2009;70:1502–11.

10. Cole TL, Center SA, Flood SN, et al. Diagnostic comparison of needle and wedge biopsy specimens of the liver in dogs and cats. J Am Vet Med Assoc 2002;220:1483–90.

11. Petre SL, McClaran JK, Bergman PJ, et al. Safety and efficacy of laparoscopic hepatic biopsy in dogs: 80 cases (2004-2009). J Am Vet Med Assoc 2012;240:181–5.

12. Rawlings CA, Howerth EW. Obtaining quality biopsies of the liver and kidney. J Am Anim Hosp Assoc 2004;40:352–8.

13. Cuddy LC, Risselada M, Ellison GW. Clinical evaluation of a pre-tied ligating loop for liver biopsy and liver lobectomy. J Small Anim Pract 2013;54:61–6.

14. Schwarz LA, Penninck DG, Leveille-Webster C. Hepatic abscesses in 13 dogs: a review of the ultrasonographic findings, clinical data and therapeutic options. Vet Radiol Ultrasound 1998;39(4):357–65.

15. Sergeeff JS, Armstrong PJ, Bunch SE. Hepatic abscesses in cats: 14 cases (1985-2002). J Vet Intern Med 2004;18:295–300.

16. van Sprundel RG, van den Ingh TS, Guscetti F, et al. Classification of primary hepatic tumours in the dog. Vet J 2013;197(3):596–606.

17. Steen S, Conway C, Guerra C, et al. 90% hepatectomy with a porto-hepatic shunt in a canine model: a feasibility study. ILAR J 2012;53(1):E1–8.

18. May LR, Mehler SJ. Complications of hepatic surgery in companion animals. Vet Clin North Am Small Anim Pract 2011;51(5):935–48.

19. Mehler SJ. Complications of the extrahepatic biliary surgery in companion animals. Vet Clin North Am Small Anim Pract 2011;51(5):949–67.

20. Head LL, Daniel GB. Correlation between hepatobiliary scintigraphy and surgery or postmortem examination findings in dogs and cats with extrahepatic biliary obstruction, partial obstruction, or patency of the biliary system: 18 cases (1995-2004). J Am Vet Med Assoc 2005;227:1618–24.

21. Huang Q, Liu CH, Zhu CL, et al. The choice of surgical timing for biliary duct reconstruction after obstructive bile duct injury: an experimental study. Hepato-gastroenterology 2013;60(128):1865–72.

22. Baker SG, Mayhew PD, Mehler SJ. Choledochotomy and primary repair of extra-hepatic biliary duct rupture in seven dogs and two cats. J Small Anim Pract 2011;52:32–7.

23. Geng L, Luo D, Zhang HC, et al. Microvessel density at different levels of normal or injured bile duct in dogs and its surgical implications. Hepatobiliary Pancreat Dis Int 2011;10:83–7.

24. Sato M, Shibata C, Kikuchi D, et al. Effects of biliary and pancreatic juice diversion into the ileum on gastrointestinal motility and gut hormone secretion in conscious dogs. Surgery 2010;148:1012–9.

25. Eich CS, Ludwig LL. The surgical treatment of cholelithiasis in cats: a study of nine cases. J Am Anim Hosp Assoc 2002;38:290–6.

26. Mayhew PD. Advanced laparoscopic procedures (hepatobiliary, endocrine) in dogs and cats. Vet Clin North Am Small Anim Pract 2009;39(5):925–39.

27. Nau P, Liu J, Ellison EC, et al. Novel reconstruction of the extrahepatic biliary tree with a biosynthetic absorbable graft. HPB (Oxford) 2011;13:573–8.

28. Shi J, Lv Y, Yu L, et al. Interest of a new biodegradable stent coated with paclitaxel on anastomotic wound healing after biliary reconstruction. Eur J Gastroenterol Hepatol 2013;25(12):1415–23.

29. Morrison S, Prostredny J, Roa D. Retrospective study of 28 cases of cholecystoduodenostomy performed using endoscopic gastrointestinal anastomosis stapling equipment. J Am Anim Hosp Assoc 2008;44(1):10–8.

30. Breznock EM. Surgical procedures of the hepatobiliary system. In: Bojrab MJ, editor. Current techniques in small animal surgery. 4th edition. Baltimore (MD): Williams & Wilkins; 1998. p. 298–308.

31. Mayhew PD, Richardson RW, Mehler SJ, et al. Choledochal tube stenting for decompression of the extrahepatic portion of the biliary tract in dogs: 13 cases (2002-2005). J Am Vet Med Assoc 2006;228(8):1209–14.

32. Son TT, Thompson L, Serrano S, et al. Surgical intervention in the management of severe acute pancreatitis in cats: 8 cases (2003-2007). J Vet Emerg Crit Care 2010;20(4):426–35.

33. Papazoglou L, Mann FA, Wagner-Mann C. Long-term survival of dogs after cholecystoenterostomy: a retrospective study of 15 cases (1981-2005). J Am Anim Hosp Assoc 2008;44:67–74.

34. Center SA. Disease of the gallbladder and biliary tree. Vet Clin North Am Small Anim Pract 2009;39(3):543–98.

35. Burns BR, Hofmeister EH, Brainard BM. Anesthetic complications in dogs undergoing hepatic surgery: cholecystectomy *versus* non-cholecystectomy. Vet Anaesth Analg 2014;41:186–90.

Current Concepts in Congenital Portosystemic Shunts

 CrossMark

Kelley M. Thieman Mankin, DVM, MS, DACVS-SA

KEYWORDS

- Shunt • Extrahepatic • Intrahepatic • Surgical management • Embolization

KEY POINTS

- Protein C level testing may be a useful blood test to indicate liver dysfunction.
- Many methods of diagnostic imaging are available, including ultrasonography, nuclear scintigraphy, CT angiography, and MR angiography.
- Commonly performed open surgical procedures for congenital portosystemic shunt (CPSS) include the placement of ameroid constrictors or cellophane bands.
- Less invasive options for the treatment of intrahepatic and extrahepatic CPSS include laparoscopic placement of cellophane bands and interventional radiologic techniques such as coil embolization.

INTRODUCTION

This article focuses on current concepts in portosystemic shunts. A thorough review of portosystemic vascular anomalies was published in 2009.[1] Recent information on portosystemic shunts is presented.

Congenital portosystemic shunts (CPSS) are vascular anomalies that occur secondary to inappropriate closure of different portions of fetal vasculature, resulting in intrahepatic or extrahepatic CPSS. Typically, a single CPSS is present, although multiple CPSS have been reported.[2] The presence of a CPSS allows portal blood to bypass the liver and enter the systemic circulation. Operative intervention is often recommended with the goal being slow closure of the anomalous vessel to gradually accustom the liver to increased blood flow and prevent the development of portal hypertension. This goal is often accomplished through open surgical techniques, including ameroid constrictor or cellophane band placement. These surgical procedures should result in CPSS closure over approximately 2 to 5 weeks and good clinical results. More

The author has nothing to disclose.
Department of Small Animal Clinical Sciences, College of Veterinary Medicine and Biomedical Sciences, Texas A&M University, 4474 TAMU, College Station, TX 77843-4474, USA
E-mail address: KThieman@CVM.tamu.edu

Vet Clin Small Anim 45 (2015) 477–487
http://dx.doi.org/10.1016/j.cvsm.2015.01.008

recently, minimally invasive methods of CPSS occlusion have been described.[3–8] Laparoscopic placement of cellophane bands has been described in dogs with extrahepatic CPSS, and endovascular occlusion has been described in dogs with either intrahepatic or extrahepatic CPSS.[3]

DIAGNOSTICS

Diagnosis and treatment of CPSS in dogs has evolved with technology. Although some aspects of the diagnostic workup and treatment of CPSS have remained similar for several years, other aspects have changed dramatically.

Clinicopathologic Findings

Laboratory testing is among the first steps recommended in the diagnostic workup of dogs suspected to have CPSS. A complete blood count (CBC), serum biochemistry profile, urinalysis, and preprandial and postprandial serum bile acids, and/or ammonia level are recommended. Recently, some veterinarians have begun testing protein C activity.

Protein C is a plasma anticoagulation protein. Along with antithrombin, protein S, and plasminogen, protein C is important for preventing thromboembolic disease. Protein C is a vitamin K–dependent serine protease enzyme that is synthesized by the liver. Once activated, protein C works to promote fibrinolysis, modulate inflammation, and inhibit apoptosis. In human patients, measurement of protein C levels has been used to assess liver function. Low protein C activity levels have been reported in people with a variety of liver diseases including inflammatory hepatopathy, cirrhosis, portal vein obstruction, and neoplastic infiltration.[9,10] Protein C activity levels may be used to assess hepatic function in a variety of liver diseases. In dogs, protein C may be useful in distinguishing CPSS from portal vein hypoplasia (also known as microvascular dysplasia).[11] Dogs with CPSS have significantly lower protein C activities than dogs with portal vein hypoplasia.[11] When protein C activity is considered with other laboratory findings, it may be useful to distinguish CPSS from portal vein hypoplasia. Further, dogs surgically treated for CPSS show postoperative improvement in protein C activity. Therefore, protein C activity levels may be a useful test, in addition to other blood tests, to aid in monitoring dogs after surgical treatment of CPSS.[11]

In humans, inflammation has been shown to be associated with hepatic encephalopathy (HE). For that reason, markers of inflammation, such as C-reactive protein, have been measured in dogs with CPSS.[12] A difference in C-reactive protein concentrations has been detected between dogs with CPSS exhibiting HE versus those not exhibiting HE and dogs without HE.[12]

Abnormalities in the CBC and serum biochemistry profile may be seen in dogs with CPSS. Changes in the CBC may include leukocytosis, microcytosis, and normocytic, normochromic, nonregenerative anemia. Leukocytosis may be present owing to increased antigenic stimulation from decreased hepatic endotoxin and bacterial clearance from the portal circulation. Anemia is seen commonly in dogs with CPSS and is associated with abnormalities in iron metabolism. The exact pathogenesis of CPSS-associated anemia has not been described. Recently, 1 study evaluated CPSS-associated anemia with abnormalities in hepcidin. Hepcidin is a hormone synthesized mainly by hepatocytes. It controls iron transport by binding and inhibiting ferroportin, an iron export protein. No evidence that dysregulated production of hepcidin was associated with anemia in dogs with CPSS was found.[13]

Changes seen on serum biochemistry profile are varied and may include decreased blood urea nitrogen, hypoalbuminemia, hypoglycemia, and hypocholesterolemia.

Other abnormalities may include mild to moderate increases in serum liver enzyme activities. Determination of either bile acids and/or baseline ammonia level should be performed on dogs with suspected CPSS. Baseline ammonia level testing in fasting animals is nearly 100% sensitive, and ammonia tolerance testing is rarely necessary.[1,14]

Abnormalities in trace minerals also may be recognized. Manganese levels have been shown to be higher in dogs with CPSS than in healthy dogs or dogs with nonhepatic illness.[15] Manganese toxicity in humans and animals results in psychiatric disturbances, gait abnormalities, and cognitive deficits; therefore, elevated manganese levels may play a role in CPSS-associated HE.[15]

Diagnostic Imaging

Intraoperative mesenteric portography

Historically, intraoperative mesenteric portography was performed frequently to diagnose CPSS. This diagnostic modality is highly invasive but sensitive.[1] Findings on intraoperative mesenteric portography may be predictive of outcome after attenuation of CPSS.[16] The degree of intrahepatic portal vessel opacification during intraoperative mesenteric portography correlates with the ability to completely ligate the CPSS.[16] After CPSS occlusion, the degree of intrahepatic portal vascular opacification was greater in dogs without encephalopathy and in dogs with postoperative clinical improvement.[16] Another benefit of portovenography is the opportunity to measure portal venous pressures. The measurement of portal pressures may assist the surgeon in operative decision making.

Limitations of mesenteric portography include expense, difficulty in interpreting images based on patient positioning, and exposure of surgeon and staff to radiation. The major limitation of mesenteric portography is its invasive nature. Risks associated with laparotomy and general anesthesia may not be acceptable for owners, especially if a diagnosis of CPSS has not been made and the opportunity to treat concurrently is undetermined. Although this diagnostic modality may be used during laparotomy with treatment administered concurrently, the surgeon may wish to have a diagnosis before performing laparotomy. Less invasive methods (eg, abdominal ultrasonography, scintigraphy, MRI angiography, CT angiography) may be performed before surgery.

Abdominal ultrasonography

Abdominal ultrasonography is a noninvasive, accessible imaging modality that is used commonly to diagnose CPSS. Reported sensitivities and specificities associated with diagnosing CPSS using ultrasonography range from 80% to 95% and 67% to 100%, respectively.[17–20] Operator experience is important when diagnosing CPSS with abdominal ultrasonography; a marked decrease in false-negative results is reported with increasing operator experience.[18] Doppler ultrasonography has a reported sensitivity of 95% and specificity of 98%.[17] An experienced ultrasonographer may be able to determine the exact position and morphology of a CPSS. Ultrasound examination allows evaluation of the entire abdomen, including the urinary tract. Unfortunately, abdominal ultrasound examination of the abdominal vasculature is relatively time consuming and tedious.

Recently, the use of trans-splenic injection of agitated saline and heparinized blood has been evaluated to aid in the ultrasonographic diagnosis of CPSS in dogs.[21] Microbubbles are followed ultrasonographically through the portal system. Microbubbles cannot traverse the sinusoidal barrier of the liver in normal dogs; therefore, the presence of the microbubbles in the systemic circulation is the criterion used to diagnose CPSS. As described, the microbubble study is performed in a patient under mild to moderate sedation.[21] The spleen is identified by ultrasound and a needle connected to an extension tube is introduced into the splenic parenchyma. The ultrasound transducer is repositioned to follow the microbubbles through the portal system. Agitated saline mixed with 1 mL of heparinized blood is injected into the spleen. The saline mixture is administered as a bolus over approximately 3 seconds and the ultrasound transducer monitors 3 locations in the abdomen. This technique is able to differentiate between intrahepatic and extrahepatic CPSS.[21] It is also able to differentiate between portoazygos and protocaval shunts and is useful to monitor dogs postoperatively for effective shunt attenuation.[21]

Scintigraphy

A nuclear portogram can be performed either trans-splenically or per rectum. Either method enables calculation of a shunt fraction, which represents the amount of blood that flows through the shunting vessel and bypasses the liver. Trans-splenic portal scintigraphy is able to provide information about shunt number and location, and requires less radionuclide than per-rectal scintigraphy, thus improving safety and allowing earlier operative intervention.[22] Sensitivity and specificity have been reported to be 88% and 67%, respectively for per-rectal scintigraphy[23] and 100% and 100%, respectively for trans-splenic scintigraphy.[22] Although trans-splenic portal scintigraphy has greater sensitivity and specificity and other benefits, complications can occur. Injection of the radionuclide into the spleen can lead to splenic hemorrhage. Similarly, injection of the radionuclide into the spleen may be difficult in smaller animals. Ultrasound guidance is often used for injection, but the injection may still occur outside the splenic parenchyma.

Computed tomographic angiography

Computed tomographic (CT) angiography is considered the best diagnostic imaging procedure for diagnosing portosystemic shunts (PSS) in humans.[24] CT angiography is gaining in popularity for use in diagnosing CPSS in dogs. It has been shown to be both sensitive (96%) and specific (89%) in dogs.[25] It is performed rapidly, provides 3-dimensional images, is noninvasive, and can provide excellent anatomic localization of shunt origin and insertion. CT angiography was shown to be 5.5 times more likely to correctly ascertain the presence or absence of CPSS compared with abdominal ultrasonography.[25]

Magnetic resonance angiography

MRI with angiography (MRA) is sporatically utilized as a diagnostic technique for CPSS. Magnetic resonance angiography provides 3-dimensional imaging of the shunt in good to excellent detail.[26] The exact anatomic position of the CPSS should be determined easily by MRA. Unfortunately, MRA can be time consuming and expensive. Reportedly, sensitivity and specificity of MRA for diagnosis of a single congenital shunt are 79% and 100%, respectively.[27] Although MRA is a promising new diagnostic modality for diagnosis of CPSS, CT angiography provides similar detail, is performed more quickly, and is often less expensive than MRA.

TREATMENT OF CONGENITAL PORTOSYSTEMIC SHUNTS

Surgical and medical treatments are available for dogs with CPSS. The goal of surgical treatment is to occlude blood flow through the shunt, thus directing portal blood through the available portal vasculature. The goal of medical management is to decrease the transport of factors absorbed from the gastrointestinal tract to the systemic circulation. One focus of medical management is reduction of ammonia absorption and systemic circulation. Both medical and surgical management play a role in the treatment of dogs with CPSS and are often used in combination. A study found that the probability of survival for dogs with CPSS receiving medical treatment alone was lower than the probability of survival for dogs receiving surgical treatment.[28] A review of medical management of CPSS can be found elsewhere.[1]

Surgical treatment of CPSS in dogs and cats has evolved in the last 10 years. Most commonly used surgical options for attenuation of CPSS include placement of an ameroid constrictor (Research Instruments N.W., Inc, Lebanon, OR; researchinstrumentsnw.com) or cellophane band. Other minimally invasive options for identification and attenuation of CPSS include laparoscopy or interventional radiology.[1]

Preoperative Management

Proper patient management is appropriate before CPSS attenuation by ameroid constrictor or cellophane banding. Such management usually includes diagnostic workup and preoperative medical treatment. Once a diagnosis of CPSS has been made, medical therapy is usually instituted. Many surgeons recommend medical management of the CPSS patient to alleviate signs of HE before surgery, presumably to decrease blood ammonia levels and create a more stable anesthetic and surgical candidate. Preoperative medical management often consists of administration of oral lactulose, neomycin (or other non–orally absorbed antimicrobial), low-protein diet, and possibly anticonvulsant medication. One study has shown pretreatment with levetiracetam to be beneficial in preventing postoperative seizures.[29] Pretreatment with levetiracetam is instituted at least 24 hours before surgery and administered at 20 mg/kg by mouth every 8 hours. The study reports that no dogs pretreated with levetiracetam experienced postoperative seizures and 5% of dogs not treated with levetiracetam experienced postoperative seizures. All the dogs in this study underwent surgery for attenuation of an extrahepatic CPSS by ameroid ring constrictor placement.[29] Some surgeons elect to start proton pump inhibitors before surgical intervention, particularly for occlusion of intrahepatic CPSS.[1]

During the pretreatment period, the animal is prepared for surgery. Such preparation includes a preoperative fast, although a 12-hour fast in small patients with CPSS is not advised owing to the potential for hypoglycemia. Dextrose-containing fluids may be indicated to prevent hypoglycemia. Additionally, a small amount of easily digestible food may be administered until 4 to 6 hours preoperatively. Regardless, when fasting is instituted, the dog should be monitored for clinical signs of hypoglycemia and treated if appropriate.

Before and after induction of general anesthesia, monitor the patient for hypoproteinemia, hypotension, hypothermia, and hypoglycemia. Hypoproteinemia is common in dogs with CPSS. Depending on the severity of hypoproteinemia, colloidal support may be indicated. Hypotension and hypothermia are also common and are a serious concern for the anesthetic team.

Technique/Procedure

Open operative technique

With ameroid constrictor or cellophane band placement through a routine celiotomy, position the patient in dorsal recumbency, and perform a ventral midline abdominal approach. Take care while opening the abdomen to not transect a CPSS within the falciform fat. Identify the anomalous vessel. Different anatomic descriptions have been made for extrahepatic CPSS. Historically, CPSS have been categorized as either portoazygos or portocaval. Introduction of more advanced diagnostic imaging techniques (eg, MRA, CT angiography) has allowed more specific characterization of 6 types of CPSS: splenocaval, splenoazygos, splenophrenic, right gastric–caval, right gastric–caval with caudal shunt loop, and right gastric–azygos with caudal shunt loop.[30] Splenophrenic and right gastric-azygos shunt with caudal loop are newly described anatomic variants of CPSS.[30] Splenophrenic shunts originate from the splenic vein and pass cranial to the liver to terminate in the caudal vena cava.[30] The right gastric–azygos shunt with caudal loop seems to have a component of right gastric–azygos and splenoazygos shunts, and it is likely that the right gastric vein is the dominant contributor to the shunting blood.[30]

Surgical treatment of all types of CPSS is similar when applying a cellophane band or ameroid constrictor. Identify the portal vein, because some dogs have portal agenesis or atresia, making attenuation of CPSS contraindicated. Inspect the caudal vena cava to identify the anomalous vessel. This process is usually accomplished by direct inspection of the vasculature, although intraoperative mesenteric portography may be performed occasionally. No large veins normally enter the caudal vena cava between the renal and hepatic veins. A shunt entering the caudal vena cava often produces turbulent blood flow with dilation of the caudal vena cava. These features may assist in the detection of the shunt. Inspect the area of the epiploic foramen. Also inspect other potential locations of extrahepatic CPSS, because multiple congenital CPSS may be present.[2] Other reported locations for CPSS include the falciform fat, gastrophrenic extrahepatic portocaval shunt, caudal abdominal CPSS, and portoazygous shunts. Gastrophrenic shunts are identified near the lesser curvature of the stomach, joining the phrenic vein at the level of the diaphragm. Caudal abdominal CPSS enter the caudal vena cava caudal to the renal veins. Portoazygous shunts cross the diaphragm and are found most commonly at the aortic or esophageal hiatus.

Place the occluding device (ameroid or cellophane band) as close to the caudal vena cava or diaphragm as possible. Create a small window in the tissues surrounding the shunt, and place the ameroid constrictor or cellophane band around the shunting vessel. Select an ameroid constrictor such that the internal diameter of the constrictor is equal to or slightly larger than the CPSS. With a cellophane band, fold the segment of cellophane in thirds longitudinally and pass it around the shunt. Loop the cellophane band back on itself, creating a ring around the CPSS. Compress the CPSS to a diameter of 3.0 mm or less with the cellophane band.[31] Alternatively, placement of the cellophane band without CPSS occlusion has been shown to be effective.[32] Secure the ends of the cellophane band together with hemoclips in an alternating pattern.[33] Placement of the constrictor as distal on the shunting vessel as possible enables inclusion of all shunt tributaries. Minimal dissection around the CPSS provides some stability to the ameroid constrictor or cellophane band to help prevent twisting or kinking of the shunting vessel.

Overall, the use of ameroid constrictors and cellophane bands for attenuation of extrahepatic CPSS results in good outcomes.[34] Long-term clinical outcomes for 206 dogs with an extrahepatic CPSS treated with an ameroid constrictor revealed that 7% of the dogs died within a month of surgery, 24% had continued shunting, and 92% had no clinical signs. Overall, 75% of dogs had successful outcomes, with 25% having unsuccessful outcomes. The median survival time was 153 months. In 22 dogs with extrahepatic CPSS treated by ameroid ring placement, CT angiography at least 8 weeks postoperatively revealed that, although none of the ameroid constrictors closed completely, only 18% of dogs had residual shunt flow.[35] Owners of dogs with residual flow reported no impact on the clinical condition of the dog, and reoperation was not recommended.

Testing of mechanical properties of cellophane film commonly used for banding CPSS revealed that only 1 of 4 films was cellophane.[36] Saline immersion and 3 methods of sterilization (ethylene oxide, gamma irradiation, and hydrogen peroxide) decreased the strength of the cellophane bands.[36] Only autoclave sterilization did not weaken the wet cellophane.[36]

Minimally invasive technique

Vessel attenuation devices can be placed in patients with congenital extrahepatic CPSS by minimally invasive techniques, including laparoscopy and interventional radiology. The technique for laparoscopic surgery is similar to that described for placement of a cellophane band in an open surgical technique. Place the first scope portal just caudal to the umbilicus. Place 2 instrument portals (to the left and right) caudal to the first portal. Place 2 sutures through the body wall and into the ventral stomach to retract the stomach and improve visibility. Inspect the epiploic foramen and other areas in the description carefully. Dissect the CPSS from the surrounding tissues. Prepare a strip of cellophane by folding it longitudinally and securing each end to a piece of silk suture. Pass the cellophane into the abdomen and place it around the CPSS with the help of the silk sutures. Secure the cellophane with hemoclips placed in an alternating pattern while lifting the attached silk sutures. A more detailed description of laparoscopic placement of cellophane bands for attenuation of a CPSS is available.[3]

Interventional radiologic methods, using fluoroscopy, can be used to attenuate CPSS. Only a small incision is made to allow access to the vasculature (eg, femoral, saphenous, jugular vein) for introduction of instruments and implements.

Although interventional radiology is used more often in dogs with intrahepatic CPSS, it can also be used in dogs with extrahepatic CPSS.[4] The Amplatzer vascular plug has been used to achieve acute occlusion of the CPSS. To assess tolerance to complete occlusion of the CPSS, monitor heart rate and systemic arterial blood pressure during complete, temporary occlusion of the CPSS. An increase in heart rate or decrease in systemic arterial blood pressure during complete temporary occlusion of the CPSS was interpreted as the patient's intolerance of complete occlusion owing to portal hypertension. Only 1 of 7 dogs in the study was intolerant to acute occlusion.[4] No complications were observed in 6 dogs acutely occluded by an Amplatzer vascular plug.[4]

Coils have been used to attenuate blood flow through the CPSS.[5–7] Coil migration was more likely to occur in dogs with extrahepatic versus intrahepatic CPSS when a vena caval stent was not used. The technique of coil embolization of intrahepatic CPSS has been refined, including placement of a stent in the caudal vena cava to minimize coil migration.[6] Use of a vena caval stent in the coil embolization of extrahepatic CPSS in dogs has been described.[7] Confirm shunt location by cavography, and introduce a catheter into the shunt via the CPSS. Coils are deployed into the CPSS until they occupy more than 75% of the shunt diameter. Closure of the CPSS without development of portal hypertension results in most cases.[7]

Because many intrahepatic shunts are difficult to treat with an open surgical procedure, interventional radiology techniques may provide a better option. The endovascular treatment of intrahepatic shunts in dogs resulted in an excellent, fair, or poor outcome in 66%, 15%, and 19%, respectively. Dogs with an excellent outcome had absence of clinical signs without administration of low-protein diet or medications. Fair outcomes were seen in dogs with an absence of clinical signs on a low-protein diet or medications, whereas poor outcomes were dogs with continued or worsening clinical signs despite low-protein diet or medications, lack of response to surgery, or surgery-related death.

Postoperative Treatment

Monitoring of the postoperative patient is critical after surgical management of CPSS. Dogs undergoing treatment (either by open or minimally invasive techniques) may exhibit portal hypertension, hypoglycemia, hypotension, or seizures. Portal hypertension is a serious complication and can be fatal. Monitoring for clinical signs of portal hypertension, including abdominal distension, abdominal pain, systemic hypotension, prolonged capillary refill time, pale mucous membranes, and gastrointestinal hemorrhage (usually evidenced by bloody diarrhea), is performed.[1] Mild portal hypertension resulting in ascites is often self-limiting.[1] Postoperative laboratory and imaging studies may be indicated. In the presence of severe clinical signs, disseminated intravascular coagulopathy, and hypotension unresponsive to fluid therapy, removal of the occlusion device may be required.

Hypoglycemia and hypotension are common postoperative complications. In 1 study, 44% of dogs had a blood glucose level of 60 g/dL or less postoperatively.[37] Hypoglycemia may be avoided in some cases by feeding small, frequent meals once the animal is awake from anesthesia. Additionally, intravenous administration of a dextrose solution is useful in preventing hypoglycemia. Regardless of preventative measures, blood glucose is monitored postoperatively. Monitoring for clinical signs of hypoglycemia, including lethargy, dull mentation, and seizures, is recommended. If indicated, dextrose may be administered as a bolus or added to the intravenous fluids. In some cases of refractory hypoglycemia, administration of dexamethasone (0.1–0.2 mg/kg intravenously) has been used successfully as treatment.[37] Hypotension may also occur postoperatively. Blood pressure is monitored regularly in postoperative patients, and treatment is administered if necessary. Treatment of hypotension may include administration of intravenous fluids, colloids and/or pressor drugs.

Postoperative seizures occur in 5% to 12% of dogs.[38,39] Postoperative seizures are often refractory to standard anticonvulsant drug treatment, and progress to status epilepticus.[39] Status epilepticus develops typically within 2 to 3 days postoperatively.[40] Pretreatment with levetiracetam is reported to decrease the incidence of postoperative seizures, as discussed.[29] Other treatments such as benzodiazepines, barbiturates, and propofol have been attempted with varying results.[41,42] Despite attempts at different treatments, a high mortality rate is associated with the development of postoperative status epilepticus.[38,39,42]

OUTCOMES

Dogs undergoing surgical treatment for CPSS often experience 1 of 3 long-term outcomes: closure of the shunt with improved portal blood flow, closure or partial closure of the shunt with improved portal blood flow and persistence of abnormal laboratory findings, or development of portal hypertension resulting in multiple acquired portosystemic shunts.

Ideally, surgery results in complete closure of the portosystemic shunt, resolution of clinical signs, and normalization of laboratory findings. Once the shunting vessel has been occluded, dogs experience increased liver volume,[43,44] presumably from hepatic regeneration.[45] In 1 study, all dogs undergoing surgery for CPSS attenuation had resolution of clinical signs, but 16% of dogs continued to have abnormal laboratory findings.[31]

In 18% to 21% of dogs, the portosystemic shunt does not close completely, resulting in residual blood flow.[35,38] Factors predictive of continued shunting are low preoperative plasma albumin levels, high portal pressure after complete shunt occlusion, and high portal pressure difference.[38] In dogs with persistent shunting, abnormalities in laboratory and imaging studies are present.[35,38] Residual shunting could occur secondary to failure of the primary shunt to close, or surgical error or presence of additional hepatic abnormalities.[35] Treatment recommended depends on the presence of clinical signs and the cause of residual shunting. If blood flow is present in the primary CPSS and clinical signs are present, or if an additional CPSS is identified that was missed during the first surgery, operative intervention is recommended.[1] If no blood flow is detected in the primary shunt and no additional shunts are found, a liver biopsy may be considered to diagnose portal vein hypoplasia.

An additional cause of shunting in a postoperative dog is the development of multiple acquired PSS. Multiple acquired PSS may occur in nearly 10% to 20% of cases undergoing surgical treatment for a single CPSS and occur when the liver is unable to tolerate increased portal blood flow.[46] Such vessels open in response to elevated portal pressures. Treatment is focused on controlling clinical signs of HE and slowing progression of the liver disease.[1]

SUMMARY

Protein C level testing may be a useful blood test to indicate liver dysfunction. Many methods of diagnostic imaging are available including ultrasound, nuclear scintigraphy, CT angiography, and MRA. Commonly performed open surgical procedures for CPSS include the placement of ameroid constrictors or cellophane bands. Less invasive options are available for the treatment of both intrahepatic and extrahepatic CPSS and include laparoscopic placement of cellophane bands and interventional radiology techniques, such as coil embolization.

REFERENCES

1. Berent AC, Tobias KM. Portosystemic vascular anomalies. Vet Clin North Am Small Anim Pract 2009;39:514–41.
2. Leeman JJ, Kim SE, Reese DJ, et al. Multiple congenital PSS in a dog: case report and literature review. J Am Anim Hosp Assoc 2013;49:281–5.
3. Miller NA. Laparoscopy: laparoscopic extrahepatic portosystemic shunt attenuation. In: Tams TR, Rawlings CA, editors. Small animal endoscopy. 3rd edition. St Louis (MO): Elsevier; 2011. p. 446–9.
4. Hogan DF, Benitez ME, Parnell NK, et al. Intravascular occlusion for the correction of extrahepatic portosystemic shunts in dogs. J Vet Intern Med 2010;25: 1048–54.
5. Leveille R, Johnson SE, Birchard SJ. Transvenous coil embolization of portosystemic shunt in dogs. Vet Radiol Ultrasound 2003;44:32–6.
6. Gonzalo-Orden JM, Altonaga JR, Costilla S, et al. Transvenous coil embolization of an intrahepatic portosystemic shunt in a dog. Vet Radiol Ultrasound 2000;41: 516–8.
7. Bussadori R, Bussadori C, Millan L, et al. Transvenous coil embolization for the treatment of single congenital portosystemic shunts in six dogs. Vet J 2008; 176:221–6.
8. Weisse C, Berent AC, Todd K, et al. Endovascular evaluation and treatment of intrahepatic portosystemic shunts in dogs: 100 cases (2001–2011). J Am Vet Med Assoc 2014;244:78–94.
9. Saray A, Mesihovic R, Vanis N, et al. Clinical significance of haemostatic tests in chronic liver disease. Med Arch 2012;66:231–5.
10. Alkim H, Ayaz S, Sasmaz N, et al. Hemostatic abnormalities in cirrhosis and tumor-related portal vein thrombosis. Clin Appl Thromb Hemost 2012;18:409–15.
11. Toulza O, Center SA, Brooks MB, et al. Evaluation of plasma protein C activity for detection of hepatobiliary disease and portosystemic shunting in dogs. J Am Vet Med Assoc 2006;229:1761–71.

12. Gow AG, Marques AI, Yool DA, et al. Dogs with congenital porto-systemic shunting (cPSS) and hepatic encephalopathy have higher serum concentrations of C-reactive protein than asymptomatic dogs with cPSS. Metab Brain Dis 2012;27:227–9.

13. Frowde PE, Gow AG, Burton CA, et al. Hepatic hepcidin gene expression in dogs with a congenital portosystemic shunt. J Vet Intern Med 2014;28(4):1203–5.

14. Sterczer A, Meyer HP, Boswijk HC, et al. Evaluation of ammonia measurements in dogs with two analysers for use in veterinary practice. Vet Rec 1999;144:23–6.

15. Gow AG, Marques AI, Yool DA. Whole blood manganese concentrations in dogs with congenital portosystemic shunts. J Vet Intern Med 2010;24(1):90–6.

16. Lee KC, Lipscomb VJ, Lamb CR, et al. Association of portovenographic findings with outcome in dogs receiving surgical treatment for single congenital portosystemic shunts: 45 cases (2000–2004). J Am Vet Med Assoc 2006;229(7):1122–9.

17. Lamb CR. Ultrasonographic diagnosis of congenital portosystemic shunts in dogs: results of a prospective study. Vet Radiol Ultrasound 1996;37:281–8.

18. Holt DE, Schelling CG, Suanders HM, et al. Correlation of ultrasonographic findings with surgical, portographic, and necropsy findings in dogs and cats with portosystemic shunts (1987–1993). J Am Vet Med Assoc 1995;207:1190–3.

19. Winkler JT, Bohling MW, Tillson DM, et al. Portosystemic shunts: diagnosis, prognosis and treatment of 64 cases (1993–2001). J Am Anim Hosp Assoc 2003;39:169–85.

20. d'Anjou M, Penninck D, Cornejo L, et al. Ultrasonographic diagnosis of portosystemic shunting in dogs and cats. Vet Radiol Ultrasound 2004;45:424–37.

21. Gomez-Ochoa P, Llabres-Diaz F, Ruiz S, et al. Use of transsplenic injection of agitated saline and heparinized blood for the ultrasonographic diagnosis of macroscopic portosystemic shunts in dogs. Vet Radiol Ultrasound 2010;52:103–6.

22. Sura PA, Tobias KM, Morandi F, et al. Comparison of 99mTcO4- trans-splenic portal scintigraphy with per-rectal portal scintigraphy for diagnosis of portosystemic shunts in dogs. Vet Surg 2007;36:654–60.

23. Koblik PD, Hornof WJ. Transcolonic sodium pertechnetate Tc99m scintigraphy for diagnosis of macrovascular portosystemic shunts in dogs, cats, and potbellied pigs: 176 cases (1988–1992). J Am Vet Med Assoc 1995;207:729–33.

24. Henseler KP, Pozniak MA, Lee FT, et al. Three-dimensional CT angiography of spontaneous portosystemic shunts. Radiographics 2001;21:691–704.

25. Kim SE, Giglio RF, Reese DJ, et al. Comparison of computed tomographic angiography and ultrasonography for the detection and characterization of portosystemic shunts in dogs. Vet Radiol Ultrasound 2013;54:569–74.

26. Mai W, Weisse C. Contrast-enhanced portal magnetic resonance angiography in dogs with suspected congenital portal vascular anomalies. Vet Radiol Ultrasound 2010;52:284–8.

27. Seguin B, Tobias KM, Gavin PR, et al. Use of magnetic resonance angiography for diagnosis of portosystemic shunts in dogs. Vet Radiol Ultrasound 1999;40:251–8.

28. Greenhalgh SN, Dunning MD, McKinley TJ, et al. Comparison of survival after surgical or medical treatment in dogs with a congenital portosystemic shunt. J Am Vet Med Assoc 2010;236:1215–20.

29. Fryer KJ, Levine JM, Peycke LE, et al. Incidence of postoperative seizures with and without levetiracetam pretreatment in dogs undergoing portosystemic shunt attenuation. J Vet Intern Med 2011;25:1379–84.

30. Nelson NC, Nelson LL. Anatomy of extrahepatic portosystemic shunts in dogs as determined by computed tomography angiography. Vet Radiol Ultrasound 2011; 52:498–506.

31. Hunt GB. Effect of breed on anatomy of portosystemic shunts resulting from congenital diseases in dogs and cats: a review of 242 cases. Aust Vet J 2004; 82:746–9.

32. Frankel D, Seim H, MacPhail C, et al. Evaluation of cellophane banding with and without intraoperative attenuation for treatment of congenital extrahepatic portosystemic shunts in dogs. J Am Vet Med Assoc 2006;228:1355–60.

33. McAlinden AB, Buckley CT, Kirby BM. Biomechanical evaluation of different numbers, sizes and placement configurations of ligaclips required to secure cellophane bands. Vet Surg 2010;39:59–64.

34. Falls EL, Milovancev M, Hunt GB, et al. Long-term outcome after surgical ameroid ring constrictor placement for treatment of single extrahepatic portosystemic shunts in dogs. Vet Surg 2013;42:951–7.

35. Hunt GB, Culp WT, Mayhew KN, et al. Evaluation of in vivo behavior of ameroid ring constrictors in dogs with congenital extrahepatic portosystemic shunts using computed tomography. Vet Surg 2014;43(7):834–42.

36. Smith RR, Hunt GB, Garcia-Nolen TC, et al. Spectroscopic and mechanical evaluation of thin film commonly used for banding congenital portosystemic shunts in dogs. Vet Surg 2013;42:478–87.

37. Holford AL, Tobias KM, Bartges JW, et al. Adrenal response to adrenocorticotropic hormone in dogs before and after surgical attenuation of a single congenital portosystemic shunt. J Vet Intern Med 2008;22:832–8.

38. Mehl ML, Kyles AE, Hardie EM, et al. Evaluation of ameroid ring constrictors for treatment for single extrahepatic portosystmic shunts in dogs: 168 cases (1995–2001). J Am Vet Med Assoc 2005;226:2020–30.

39. Tisdall PL, Hunt GB, Youmans KR, et al. Neurological dysfunction in dogs following attenuation of congenital extrahepatic portosystemic shunts. J Small Anim Pract 2000;41:539–46.

40. Fossum TW. Surgery of the liver. In: Fossum TW, editor. Small animal surgery textbook. 3rd edition. St Louis (MO): Mosby Elsevier; 2007. p. 531–60.

41. Gommeren K, Claeys S, de Rooster H, et al. Outcome from status epilepticus after portosystemic shunt attenuation in 3 dogs treated with propofol and phenobarbital. J Vet Emerg Crit Care (San Antonio) 2010;20:346–51.

42. Heldmann E, Holt DE, Brockman DJ, et al. Use of propofol to manage seizure activity after surgical treatment of portosystemic shunts. J Small Anim Pract 1999;40:590–4.

43. Stieger SM, Zwingenberger A, Pollard RE, et al. Hepatic volume estimation using quantitative computed tomography in dogs with portosystemic shunts. Vet Radiol Ultrasound 2007;48:409–13.

44. Kummeling A, Vrakking DJ, Rothuizen J, et al. Hepatic volume measurements in dogs with extrahepatic congenital portosystemic shunts before and after surgical attenuation. J Vet Intern Med 2010;24:114–9.

45. Tivers MS, Lipscomb VJ, Smith KC, et al. Markers of hepatic regeneration associated with surgical attenuation of congenital portosystemic shunts in dogs. Vet J 2014;200:305–11.

46. Matthews KG, Bunch SK. Vascular liver diseases. In: Ettinger SJ, Feldman ED, editors. Textbook of veterinary internal medicine: diseases of the dog and cat. 6th edition. St Louis (MO): Elsevier Saunders; 2005. p. 1453–64.

Thoracic Surgery; Important Considerations and Practical Steps

 CrossMark

D. Michael Tillson, DVM, MS

KEYWORDS

- Thoracic surgery • Thoracotomy • Sternotomy • Trandsdiaphragmatic thoracotomy
- Thoracostomy tube • Thoracic anatomy

KEY POINTS

- Outcomes associated with thoracic surgery are related more to the underlying disease process than the surgical approach.
- Straightforward surgical procedures including vascular surgeries have excellent outcomes, whereas more complex procedures tend to have less positive outcomes.
- Investment in facilities and equipment is needed to properly perform thoracic surgery. Reluctance to make this investment seemingly reduces the effectiveness of the surgeon and decreases the likelihood of a successful outcome.

Surgical skills required for performing a thoracotomy are not particularly different than those used for other surgeries, although there are some specific skills to be considered. Challenges of performing a thoracotomy include a lack of familiarity with procedures, concerns about perioperative and anesthesia management, need for 24-hour monitoring after surgery and decision-making steps required for a successful procedure and outcome.

Performing successful thoracic surgery is feasible for an experienced general surgeon in a well-equipped practice. This article reviews the basics of getting into and out of the thoracic cavity using standard open surgical approaches. Additionally, a template is offered to help decide whether thoracic surgical procedures are appropriate for your practice.

GENERAL OVERVIEW

This article reviews techniques and tips found useful by the author when performing thoracic surgery.

Disclosure: The author has nothing to disclose.
Department of Clinical Sciences, Bailey Small Animal Teaching Hospital, College of Veterinary Medicine, Auburn University, 1220 Wire Road, Auburn, AL 36849, USA
E-mail address: tillsdm@auburn.edu

http://dx.doi.org/10.1016/j.cvsm.2015.01.007
0195-5616/15/$ – see front matter
vetsmall.theclinics.com

Veterinary articles, in an attempt maximize sample sizes, often look at every thoracic surgery performed at a particular location by numerous individuals at various levels of training,[1–4] whereas a retrospective human study will be able to describe 600 children undergoing median sternotomy for a few, specific cardiac procedures.[5] Such veterinary studies, although often the best available, introduce several variables requiring the reader to be more discerning in their take-home message. Below are some important retrospective reviews of veterinary thoracic surgery and some of the key findings. Readers are encouraged to review the articles for additional insights.

- A review of more than 180 thoracotomies in dogs and cats showed a 78% overall survival rate.[1]
  - The most common thoracic procedures in this study were patent ductus arteriosus (PDA) ligation, diaphragmatic hernia (DH) repair and esophageal foreign body retrieval in dogs, and DH repair and thoracic exploratory surgeries for cats with pleural effusions.
  - Mortality rates after thoracotomy were found to be variable with those having a high survival rate (>90%; eg, PDA, thoracic wall trauma, congenital DH), intermediate survival rate (60%–75%; eg, persistent right aortic arch (PRAA), pulmonic stenosis, pleural effusions), and lower survival rates (<60%; eg, cardiac, pericardial, and esophageal surgeries).
  - The lowest survival rates were reported for procedures involving the great vessels and pulmonary or mediastinal tumors.
- A review reported on lateral thoracotomy in 83 small animals.[2] They found survival outcomes were significantly lower in cats compared with dogs (62% vs 91%) and in animals with neoplastic disease versus those with nonneoplastic conditions (60% vs 93%).
  - The underlying reasons for most lateral thoracotomy procedures were vascular procedures (ie, PDA, PRAA), and these procedures had the highest survival to discharge rates. Small animals undergoing esophageal and lobectomy procedures had lower but similar survival rates.
  - Complications associated with lateral thoracotomy included seroma and ventral edema [16/83], excessive wound inflammation [6/83], ipsilateral limb lameness [3/83], and wound discharge [3/83].
- A recent study evaluating 232 patients after thoracic surgery found that nearly 7% had pyothorax after a thoracotomy (lateral or median sternotomy).[3]
  - Risk factors identified included surgery for idiopathic chylous effusions and invasive, presurgical interventions for diagnostic, management, or therapeutic reasons, such as thoracocentesis or intrathoracic biopsy.
  - In dogs with pyothorax, diagnosis was confirmed an average of 7 days after surgery, and the ultimate mortality rate was 67%. Dogs with the diagnosis of chylous effusion accounted for 60% of dogs that had postoperative pyothorax.
  - The breakdown of procedures showed the most common approach was a lateral thoracotomy (67%) with median sternotomy being performed in 27% of patients. Other approaches were thoracoscopy (3%), transdiaphragmatic sternotomy (2%), or a combined transdiaphragmatic and median sternotomy (1%).
- A review of 286 dogs undergoing thoracotomy looked at factors associated with nonsurvival at 24 hours and before discharge.[4]
  - The use of neuromuscular blocking agents and the need for presurgical oxygen supplementation were risk factors for nonsurvival at 24 hours.

○ Factors identified for nonsurvival to discharge included intraoperative use of a blood product and increasing surgical duration. These factors were also attributed to more complex and complicated surgical procedures.

PERIOPERATIVE PLANNING

The first consideration before a thoracic procedure is the facility and its associated goals. A large, dedicated surgery room with high-quality and adjustable lighting is appropriate. Anesthesia equipment able to provide for either manual or mechanical ventilation of the patient and routine monitoring equipment (electrocardiogram monitor, oxygen saturation by pulse oximetry, and end-tidal CO_2 monitors) is necessary. Adequate support personnel to perform and monitor anesthesia are important. Manual ventilation requires a dedicated technician, whereas mechanical ventilation requires the availability of a trained individual to run and trouble shoot the equipment. Appropriate surgical equipment, including an electrosurgical unit and effective vacuum/suction is needed. Specific surgical instrumentation is determined by the nature of the procedure, but many routine procedures (eg, PDA ligation or routine lung lobectomy) may be accomplished with a general surgical pack and a few additional instruments (eg, Finochietto rib retractor, fine-tipped Metzenbaum scissors, and a selection of right-angle forceps). In addition, thoracic procedures require options for controlling hemorrhage, as blood loss can be significant. Appropriate instrumentation should include occluding vascular forceps of various sizes and shapes (eg, straight forceps, partial occlusion clamps, and bulldog clamps). Vascular clips of various sizes and stapling equipment help improve efficiency and can be life saving in emergency situations. Because many operative procedures in the thoracic cavity can involve the heart and great vessels, part of perioperative planning should include a realistic assessment of the need for having blood products available.

A simple technique, preplacement of Rumel tourniquets around at-risk structures or major vessels, can provide a mechanism of hemorrhage control that can influence outcome. Rumel tourniquets are created by carefully dissecting around a vessel and passing a strand of moistened umbilical tape around the vessel. The umbilical tape is passed through the lumen of a 12F to 18F red rubber catheter that was cut to a predetermined length. Hemostatic forceps (eg, Kelly) are placed on the exiting umbilical tape, and the Rumel is placed to the side of the surgical site. In the event of serious hemorrhage, the umbilical tape loop of the Rumel is tightened through the catheter segment, and the Kelly hemostat secures the tightened noose. With an appropriate-length Rumel, the surgeon can still access the surgical field to determine the reason for the hemorrhage and then attempt to fix the problem. Vessels loops (sterile, color-coded strands of soft silicon) can be used instead of umbilical tape. When making one's own Rumel tourniquets, a stiff loop of suture (eg, polypropylene) is used to catch and draw the umbilical tape through the catheter lumen. A reusable Rumel stylet can also be purchased to help draw the vessel loop through the lumen of the catheter segment.

SURGICAL APPROACHES

There are typically 3 options for open surgical approaches to the thorax in the dog and cat: a lateral (intercostal) thoracotomy created by incising on either the right or left side, median sternotomy created by incising along the ventral midline of the sternum, and transdiaphragmatic thoracotomy in which the abdominal incision allows the surgeon to incise the diaphragm to access the caudal portion of the thoracic cavity.[6–9] Minimally invasive options for thoracic procedures are discussed elsewhere in this issue by Radlinsky. The remainder of this article focuses on performing these procedures, including indications for each, examining anatomic aspects, and recounting details for getting into and out of the thoracic cavity.

LATERAL (INTERCOSTAL) THORACOTOMY
Indications

Indications for performing a lateral (intercostal) thoracotomy broadly include any situation in which there is a need to access only one hemithorax. This may include pulmonary procedures (eg, complete or partial lobectomy, mass biopsy, identification of a localized lung lesion), procedures involving the pericardium, heart, or pulmonary outflow tract, access to mediastinal, thoracic wall, or pleural structures (eg, thoracic trachea, esophagus, thoracic duct, regional lymph nodes) or lesions (eg, trauma, masses).[6,7,10]

A lateral thoracotomy typically allows for better access to structures located dorsally in the thoracic cavity (eg, pulmonary hilus, thoracic duct, bronchial lymph nodes). The size of the intercostal incision can be controlled to create a full or minithoracotomy depending on the specific needs of the procedure.

The next concern for the surgeon is deciding on the correct location for the thoracotomy incision. A lateral thoracotomy provides limited access to some structures within the thoracic cavity. Ribs on either side of the incision are the major reason for the limited access, as the ribs only can be separated by a small distance. Confirming the correct intercostal space for the incision is key when performing a lateral thoracotomy. An anatomic access chart (**Table 1**) is useful in identifying the most appropriate side and intercostal space for the surgical incision based on the target structure. The chart should be used in conjunction with imaging studies to make a final decision about the location of the intercostal incision. For pulmonary lesions, although the lesion may be located near the periphery of the lung, the targeted region to perform a pulmonary lobectomy is the hilus. The natural curvature of the ribs permits more movement by the cranial rib than the caudal rib—a slightly more caudal location (ie, fifth intercostal incision vs fourth intercostal incision) because of the potential to shift the cranial rib more significantly. Using an appropriately located incision compromised both visibility and potentially outcome.

Anatomy

Careful anatomic review before lateral thoracotomy is important. When making a lateral thoracotomy incision, the following muscles[11,12] are encountered.

- Cutaneus trunci—A thin muscle covering most of the trunk of the dog and cat. It is usually incised with the skin and subcutaneous incision.
- Latissimus dorsi—Originates from lumbodorsal fascia, which arises from the caudal thoracic and lumbar spinous processes. The muscular portion of the latissimus muscle arises from the last 2 to 3 ribs. The muscle travels cranially and inserts on the medial fascia of the brachium.
- Scalenus—Extends from the transverse processes of the cervical vertebrae (3, 4, and 5) to insertion on the fifth to eighth ribs. Because the muscular portion of the scalenus muscle terminates at the fifth rib, it can be used to help the surgeon identify the fourth intercostal side. It is normally incised during a fourth intercostal incision.
- Serratus ventralis—The thoracis portion inserts on the first 7 to 8 ribs at or slightly ventral to midline. The serrated portions are very distinct in this portion of the muscle. The serratus muscle can typically be divided along the various serrations

Table 1
Access to thoracic organs through an intercostal incision

Structure	Left	Right
Lung lobes (access to the hilus of the lung lobe)		
Left cranial	5 [6]	
Left caudal	5 [6]	
Right cranial		5 [6]
Right middle		5 [6]
Right caudal		5 [6]
Accessory		5 [6]
Heart and great vessels		
PDA, ligamentum arteriosum (PRAA)	4 [5]	
Pericardium	4 [5]	4 [5]
Pulmonary outflow tract		
Right ventricle	4 [5]	
Left ventricle	4 [5]	
Caudal vena cava	4 [5]	6 [7]
Cranial vena cava	4	4
Thymus	3 [4]	
Thoracic duct (dog)		8, 9, 10, 11
Thoracic duct (cat)	8, 9, 10, 11	
Esophagus		
Cranial (cranial to heart base)	4 [3]	3, 4, 5
Caudal (caudal to heart base)		7, 8, 9

Modified from Refs.[6,8,10]

to allow access to the intercostal muscles. Alternatively, the individual segments can be transected.

- External abdominal oblique—Originates on the fifth, sixth, and seventh ribs and can be used to help locate the fourth intercostal space.
- External intercostal—The more superficial of the intercostal muscles, the external intercostal fibers run in a craniodorsal to caudoventral direction.
- Internal intercostal—The deeper of the intercostal muscles that have fibers running in a caudodorsal to cranioventral direction. The thoracic pleural is located on its medial surface.
- Rectus abdominis—Originates from the first costal cartilages and extends ventrally to insert on the pubic brim. This muscle is generally not encountered during a routine lateral thoracotomy.

In selected situations, if there is inadequate access or visibility through the chosen intercostal incision, an adjacent rib can be removed (rib resection thoracotomy) or freed from its costal attachment to allow the rib to pivot on its dorsal articulation thereby increasing the size of the intercostal space.[13] These techniques permit greater access and easier extraction of large intrathoracic masses, but they are best used from the outset rather than trying to convert from a preexisting incision. These modifications would seem to require greater soft tissue disruption and the potential for increased hemorrhage from the intercostal vessels. As such, these modifications are not routinely used in our practice.

Approach

Once the target surgical site is determined, the hemithorax is clipped and prepared for aseptic surgery. Intercostal spaces are counted to determine the approximate location for the initial skin incision. The skin, cutaneous trunci muscle and subcutaneous tissue are incised parallel to the caudal border of the cranial rib, from dorsal to ventral and extending two-thirds of the distance from the epaxial muscles to the sternum. The latissimus dorsi muscle is incised parallel with the skin incision or retracted dorsally by freeing up the fascia along the ventral edge of the muscle.[14] Although experience suggests the dorsal retraction technique can limit the dorsal extent of the intercostal incision, it does seem to result in less postoperative lameness.

The fibers of the serratus ventralis muscle can be separated without transecting the muscle. The external and internal intercostal muscles are incised in the middle of the intercostal space. If the pleura is still intact after separating the intercostal muscles, it is incised along the same line, allowing entry into the thoracic cavity. Hemorrhage along the incision is controlled with sutures or electrosurgery.

Once the intercostal incision is complete, wound edges are covered with moistened laparotomy sponges, and a Finochietto rib spreader is inserted. The Finochietto is carefully opened to widen the intercostal space, creating access to the thoracic cavity. This process should be done slowly and deliberately to avoid excessive trauma to ribs (fracture) or the associated soft tissue, especially muscle tearing at the ventral and dorsal aspects of the intercostal incision. Furthermore, care must also be taken if the incision is continued ventrally to avoid trauma to the internal thoracic vessels. If the incision requires ventral extension, careful dissection to identify and preserve or ligate the internal thoracic vessels is appropriate.

Closure

Before lateral thoracic wall closure, sponge counts are reconciled and thoracostomy tubes are inserted and secured. Any remaining lavage fluid is aspirated from the chest cavity. Closure of a lateral thoracotomy incision is typically accomplished by preplacing multiple sutures placed in a circumcostal manner. For a fourth left intercostal incision, circumcostal suture placement incorporates ribs 4 and 5. Care is taken to avoid damaging the neurovascular bundle (ie, the intercostal artery, vein, and nerve), which courses along the caudal aspect of each rib. The underlying lung parenchyma is protected as the needle is being passed. Coordinating needle passage around the ribs with the relaxation phase of the ventilatory cycle helps decrease the risk of inadvertently damaging the underlying lung.

Circumcostal sutures are placed every 2 to 3 cm with 6 to 10 sutures used for most dogs and 5 to 8 sutures for most cats. A monofilament, absorbable suture (generally polydioxanone [PDS]) is used with suture size being appropriate for patient size.

Once all the circumcostal sutures have been preplaced, the strands are organized such that every other suture is placed on the opposite sides of the incision (**Fig. 1**). With this organization, the surgeon takes the most ventral suture (#1), and the surgical assistant grasps sutures #2 and #3 to help bring the ribs in to closer apposition while the surgeon is tying suture #1. The suture is secured with either a surgeon's knot or a slip knot. An additional 3 to 4 throws are added to ensure a secure knot. This process is continued until all sutures are tied and the ribs are apposed. Care should be taken to avoid overlapping the ribs.

Once the ribs have been apposed, the overlying soft tissue layers are apposed using an absorbable, monofilament suture, using a combination of continuous and interrupted suture patterns. Incised muscles should be accurately realigned to aid healing. The

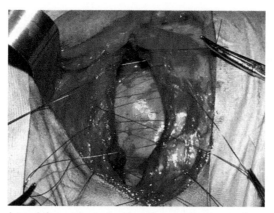

Fig. 1. Closure of a lateral thoracotomy involves the preplacement of sutures in a circumcostal manner. Sutures are placed around the rib on opposing sides of the incision. The surgeon grasps the first suture while the assistant brings the ribs into apposition using the second and third set of sutures.

subcutaneous tissues are meticulously sutured with the goal of eliminating dead space and avoiding hematoma formation. A 3-0 or 4-0, absorbable monofilament suture should be adequate for this layer. With good closure, the need for drain placement should be rare. Skin apposition is routine with staples, intradermal sutures, or skin sutures.

Technique variations relating to lateral thoracotomies are described below:

- Some surgeons prefer to bluntly dissect through the intercostal muscles into the thoracic cavity and grasp the suture with a mosquito hemostat to avoid injuring the neurovascular bundle or underlying lungs with the suture needle. Rib pivot thoracotomy is a technique to increase exposure of the thoracic cavity through a lateral thoracotomy incision.[13] For the approach, the target rib is identified, and after a standard approach to the lateral aspect of the rib, the periosteum is incised and reflected from around the rib. The rib is freed by cutting the costochondral junction, which allows the rib to pivot cranially. The medial aspect of the periosteum is incised to enter the thoracic cavity. Closure after a rib pivot thoracotomy begins with suturing the periosteum with a small, monofilament absorbable suture material and then rotating the rib back into position. A hole is drilled through the rib and adjacent cartilage and the rib is secured in position with a hemicerclage wire (20 g).
- An alternative technique has been reported for closure of a lateral thoracotomy.[15] A lateral to medial tunnel is drilled in the caudal rib, and the suture is passed through the tunnel. The suture is passed around the cranial rib in a routine manner. Less pain in the first 48 hours after surgery is observed. The basis for the technique is a cadaveric study that found that because the intercostal nerve runs along the caudal aspect of the rib, it is at risk to be encircled by circumcostal sutures and pinched against the rib. This technique could also result in iatrogenic rib fracture in small or aged animals, so careful patient selection is required.

MEDIAN STERNOTOMY
Indications

Indications for a median sternotomy are to access both sides of the thoracic cavity through a single incision, provide better access to ventral mediastinal structures, and permit thorough exploration of the thoracic cavity. Although other procedures, such as pulmonary lobectomies or thoracic duct ligations, can be accomplished through a median sternotomy, the depth of these structures from the incision can make such procedures much more challenging than they would be when using an appropriate intercostal approach. This is especially true in large dogs or deep-chested breeds.

A complication of less than 4% for median sternotomies is reported in humans, whereas a much higher complication rate (17%–70%) is reported in veterinary patients.[16–20] Reasons for this disparity may include patient differences (veterinary patients rest in sternal recumbency compared with humans), less experienced veterinary surgeons, and lack of standard agreement of what constitutes a complication in veterinary surgical studies.[17,21] Many of the outcome results in reviews of median sternotomy may be more accurately attributed to the disease process rather than to the procedure itself.

Anatomy

The canine sternum consists of 8 bones (sternebrae) separated by a short segment of cartilage (intersternebral cartilage). The first sternebrae, the manubrium, denotes the thoracic inlet, and the last sternebrae, the xiphoid, marks the cranial extent of the abdominal cavity.[11,12] Both of these sternebrae are flatter than the others, and the manubrium widens to allow the attachment of the first ribs to the bone itself. The other sternal ribs (2–9) articulate with the intersternebral cartilages found between the sternebrae themselves.[11,12,18] Intersternebral cartilages may calcify in older dogs. The remaining sternebrae are hourglass shaped with the central portion being thinner than the endplates. This conformation is dramatically different from the flatter sternum found in humans and porcine models and may predispose the sternebrae to implant-related fractures.[18] The sternum serves as the insertion point for the pectoral muscles. These muscles normally attach to the ventral and lateral surface of the sternum and rarely cross over the midline.

Procedure

A median sternotomy may be a more technically challenging surgical procedure in the dog and cat than the lateral thoracotomy. Support for the supposition that a sternotomy is inherently more problematic than a lateral thoracotomy is lacking.[21] It has been suggested that it is the fault of the underlying condition, not the approach, that is responsible for the potential bad reputation of the sternotomy.[21]

The patient should be clipped from the midpoint of the neck to the umbilicus. Laterally, the surgical site extends dorsally one-half the distance to the dorsal midline. It is important to anticipate the need for thoracostomy tubes or other drainage devices when clipping and draping the patient so potential exit sites are clipped, prepared, and draped into the sterile field. The patient is placed in dorsal recumbency and secured to minimize tilting. A tilted patient can result in the technical error of deviating too far to one side while cutting through the sternum. This can result in eccentric division of the sternebrae and greater tissue trauma and patient morbidity.

The skin and subcutaneous tissue are incised on the ventral midline along the entire length of the sternum. A Freer elevator is helpful in elevating or reflecting the sternal attachments of the pectoral muscles. Once the sternum is exposed, an oscillating saw is used to begin the sternotomy. Moderate lavage with warm saline helps prevent thermal injury to the sternebrae and keeps the incision line clear. The oscillating saw is gripped firmly in the dominant hand while the sternal cut is being performed (**Fig. 2**).

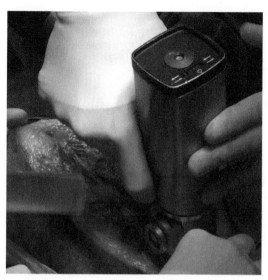

Fig. 2. An oscillating saw is held in the dominant hand while the median incision is made through the sternum. A gentle lavage is used during saw use to wash away debris and minimize thermal injury.

The nondominant hand is used to support and stabilize the saw and to prevent the saw blade from dropping into the thoracic cavity unexpectedly. Having an assistant peer down the longitudinal axis of the patient can assist the surgeon in staying on the midline and in the correct vertical orientation. The saw blade is moved along the path using a deliberate, back and forth motion.

The Freer elevator can be used to gauge depth of the sternal cut permitting the surgeon to adjust the cut as required. Before entering the thorax, the anesthesia support personnel should be told that the intrathoracic pressure is about to be equalized and that positive pressure ventilation should be initiated if not already in progress.

The current recommendation is to avoid incising the entire sternum by choosing to leave at least one end of the sternum intact (ie, the first or eighth sternebrae).[6,10,18] Although this technique may limit exposure at the undisturbed end, it does appear to prevent or minimize sternal movement (sternal shift) during the postoperative period through the maintenance of a solid point of fixation along the sternum. Sternal instability is reportedly one cause of significant discomfort in humans after sternotomy, often resulting in delayed healing and other postoperative complications.[15] Reports of delayed healing and sternal shifting as a primary complication are lacking in veterinary medicine with only a few cases of sternal fracture or osteomyelitis attributed to sternal instability.[19]

On entry, transection of some mediastinal attachments and hemorrhage control are usually necessary. Using Gelpi perineal retractors at either end of the sternotomy incision helps separate the edges of the sternum and complete the sternal incision (**Fig. 3**). The edges of the incision are covered with moistened laparotomy sponges to help prevent tissue desiccation. At this point, both sides of the thoracic cavity can be examined for whatever surgical lesion is being targeted. Appropriate samples for culture and susceptibility testing, cytology, and histopathology are taken. Adhesions are disrupted as required, all vital structures are evaluated, and the indicated surgical procedure is performed.

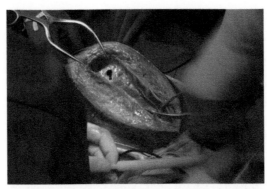

Fig. 3. Once the sternotomy incision is complete, Gelpi or Finochietto retractors can be used to spread the sternum, allowing for thoracic access. Moistened laparotomy sponges should be placed to protect the soft tissues on either side of the incision. Note that the last sternebrae was left intact to improve postoperative stability.

Sternal Closure

If appropriate, the thoracic cavity is lavaged with body temperature (100°F–103°F) isotonic saline. If a lobectomy has been performed or if there is another reason to be concerned about an air leak (eg, spontaneous pneumothorax), the entire thoracic cavity can be filled with saline and the patient ventilated to 20 cm H_2O. The saline is surveyed for evidence of air bubbles rising to the surface. If bubbles are noted, the saline is drained and the leakage addressed. Once air leaks have been controlled to the best of the surgeon's ability, the process of checking for leaks is repeated. All excessive fluid is removed from the thoracic cavity, and final checks are made, hemostasis is confirmed, and any pending samples are obtained before closure.

As with all open body cavity procedures, the preoperative and postoperative sponge count should be reconciled immediately before incision closure. Radiopaque sponges and laparotomy pads should be used for thoracic procedures, as intrathoracic procedures can be challenging. The use of radiopaque surgical sponges allows the surgeon to identify retained sponges or confirm the absence of a retained sponge, if the final sponge count does not reconcile.

Thoracostomy tube placement is best accomplished immediately before closure. The thoracostomy tube is secured to the skin with a finger trap suture before proceeding. The thoracostomy tube is left open (ie, unclamped) for the duration of the thoracic wall closure.

Most surgeons use orthopedic wire (18–22 g) in a figure-of-eight pattern to appose the cut sternebrae.[6,8,10,19,20] Various wire configurations have been evaluated with the peristernal figure-of-eight pattern being recommended (**Fig. 4**). In a porcine model, single peristernal wires or alternating peristernal and transsternal wires were rated as the most stable technique, whereas the peristernal figure-of-eight was the next best.[22] These findings are in contrast to those in a veterinary study in which a single peristernal wire (see **Fig. 4**) was found to be the least able to resist displacement forces.[23] The failure mode was sternal body fracture and attributed to the hourglass shape of the canine sternebrae. In 2 studies using a porcine model for sternotomy closure, the pericostal figure-of-eight wire was consistently inferior to other wiring methods (see **Fig. 4**).[22,24] Other materials (eg, polypropylene suture, polydioxanone suture, and nylon bands) have had varying results.[25] Sternal instability and delayed sequestrum formation were reported in 2 of 18 dogs after the sternotomy was closed

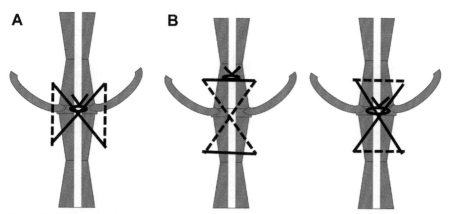

Fig. 4. Types of sternal wires. Figure-of-eight patterns are commonly used. The pericostal figure-of-eight wire configuration is shown to be less effective than the 2 versions of peri-sternal wires. (*A*) Pericostal wire placement—generally found to be less stable, not recommended. (*B*) Peristernal wire placement—Alternating the location of the twist.

using polypropylene sutures.[20] An evaluation of 4 metric (#1) polydioxanone versus stainless steel was unable to recommend polydioxanone for routine sternal closure in veterinary medicine.[26] Although suture closure has provided a secure sternal closure for the first week, it failed to maintain stability when re-evaluated at 28 days when compared with orthopedic wire.[18] Human studies and reports seem to be more focused on absorbable materials, specifically polydioxanone, for sternotomy closure in young or high-risk patients.[5,27,28] Although standard (spooled) orthopedic wire is typically used for sternal closure, use of a swagged stainless steel suture might make wire passage an easier process. The relationship between wire gauge and suture designations are presented to assist with conversion from the spooled wire to swaged-on wire sutures (**Table 2**).

All figure-of-eight wires are preplaced for sternal closure encircling the articulation between the adjacent rib and the intersternebral cartilage. Moving in a cranial to caudal direction, the tip of the wire strand is passed carefully to avoid injuring the lungs or other soft tissues (eg, internal thoracic vessel[s]). An orthopedic wire passer may prove useful, especially in larger dogs requiring a larger gauge wire in the passage of the wire strands. An alternating figure-of-eight pattern is used with the crossing wires being positioned alternatively dorsal and ventral to the sternum (**Figs. 5 and 6**). Once all the wires are placed, the sternebrae are apposed by twisting the wire. Ends are cut short, leaving 2 to 3 twists, and bent over to minimize soft tissue

Table 2
Comparison between orthopedic wire and commercial swaged, monofilament stainless steel suture

Wire (Brown & Sharpe Gauge)	Stainless Steel Suture
18 g	#7
20 g	#5
22 g	#3
24 g	#2

Steps for passing a peristernal wire for sternal closure

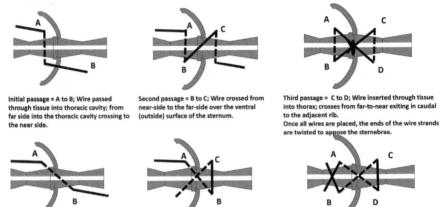

Initial passage = A to B; Wire passed through tissue into thoracic cavity; from far side into the thoracic cavity crossing to the near side.

Second passage = B to C; Wire crossed from near-side to the far-side over the ventral (outside) surface of the sternum.

Third passage = C to D; Wire inserted through tissue into thorax; crosses from far-to-near exiting in caudal to the adjacent rib.
Once all wires are placed, the ends of the wire strands are twisted to appose the sternebrae.

Fig. 5. The steps for placing peristernal figure-of-eight wires for sternal closure.

injury. Although bending over the twist the wire will have some loosening, it helps assure adequate soft tissue coverage of the wire.

Additional closure is performed in a routine manner, with an absorbable, monofilament suture material in a continuous pattern. With some patients, it may be possible to pull some of the pectoral musculature to cover the sternal incision and help with closure. Skin apposition is achieved with an intradermal pattern, skin sutures, or skin staples. Once an air-tight closure is obtained, the intrapleural pressure differential (negative thoracic pressure) can be re-established by removing residual air using the thoracostomy tube. Once a gradient of 10 to 15 cm H_2O is reached, the thoracotomy tube is clamped and secured. A chest bandage can be placed to cover the wound and secure a thoracostomy tube to the thoracic wall. Whenever a chest bandage is placed before full recovery from anesthesia, care is taken to ensure the bandage is not overly tight and compromising the patient's respiratory effects.

There should be sufficient bedding to help prevent excessive pressure along the incision line postoperatively. Wound complications associated with sternotomy may be increased through direct pressure from the patient lying on the incision. If additional padding is required, a doughnut—a buffer of bandage material on either side, but not

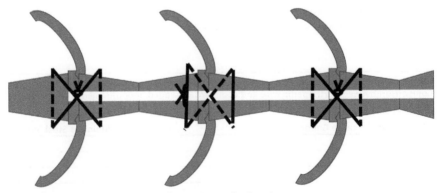

Fig. 6. The alternating technique for peristernal wire placement.

over, the incision—may be incorporated into the chest bandage. This type of chest wrap allows the patient to lay on the sternum without placing direct pressure on the incision site.

Capsular reviews for sternotomy:

- An early study found the combination of bilateral parasternal wires and transsternal wires resulted in good sternal apposition and healing. Other issues noted were wound edema, seroma, hemorrhage, and mild wound dehiscence.[29]
  - The combined wiring technique was used to minimize the potential for the transsternal wires for cutting through the thinner central sternebrae, resulting in instability and sternal dehiscence.
- Specific steps to reduce patient morbidity after sternotomy include dividing individual sternebrae along the midline and leaving 1 or 2 sternebrae intact at either end of the sternum to provide for better alignment and to minimize sternal shifting.[19]
  - The authors also recommended that sternal closure be performed with orthopedic wire (18 g or 20 g) in most dogs but open the possibility of using suture material in small dogs or cats.
- Sternotomy closure with wire compared with suture material was studied.[18]
  - Both suture closure and wire closure provided for stable sternal apposition 7 days after closure, but by 28 days after closure, the suture closure was found to be unstable in 3 of 7 (40%) dogs.
  - Although such differences were not reported to be statistically significant, from a clinical standpoint, the rate of instability seems unacceptable. Suture closure was also found to be faster than wire closure by 2.4 minutes.
- PDS suture (4 metric/#1) was compared with stainless steel wire for sternal closure in a cadaveric model. Both materials were placed in a figure-of-eight manner and distracted until failure.[25]
  - The cadaveric sternums were incised on midline, leaving the manubrium intact. Although there was no statistical difference for displacement or stiffness between the 2 materials, there was a significant difference in load to failure with the stainless steel being significantly stronger than the PDS.
  - The suture material suffered suture failure, whereas the wire failed with deformation of soft tissues or fracture of the sternebrae.
  - PDS was suggested as a viable alternative in selected patient populations, eg, pediatric, dogs with muscle wasting, osteoporotic bone, unequal sternal cuts, or dogs with prominent sternal bones.
  - It was recommended to use a slip knot for the initial knot, as manual manipulation found the surgeon's throw to have loosened.

TRANSDIAPHRAGMATIC THORACOTOMY
Indications

Transdiaphragmatic thoracotomy may be indicated in several specific circumstances. This procedure provides excellent access to the caudal thoracic duct, the caudal vena cava, the caudal portion of the esophagus, and the heart for epicardial lead placement or cardiopulmonary resuscitation.[7,8] This is the author's procedure of choice for thoracic duct ligation as a part of managing chylous effusions, allowing for a single approach for intraoperative lymphangiography and methylene blue infusion. In most situations, access to the thoracic duct is good without the need for a caudal sternotomy. Diaphragmatic incision may be useful during resection of large hepatic masses or in dissection and attenuation of large intrahepatic shunts. The transdiaphragmatic approach may also be a part of reducing herniated organs when correcting large diaphragmatic hernias.

Procedure

A standard abdominal celiotomy is used for this approach. The patient is draped to permit the extension of the incision both caudally and cranially, if required. A self-retaining retractor (Balfour-type) is placed, and the falciform ligament is removed. Having an assistant retract the cranial aspect of the abdominal incision with the Balfour spoon (or other hand-held retractor) will improve the visibility of the diaphragm. Moistened laparotomy sponges should be used to help protect the liver during retraction and exposure.

The surgeon needs to identify the correct location for the proposed diaphragmatic incision: right-side, left-side, or central. This decision is normally based on the specific needs of the procedure. Centrally located incisions may be made through the central tendinous portion of the diaphragm. Right- or left-sided approaches are made by splitting the muscular fibers in a radial direction. The incision can be continued along the circumference of the diaphragm to increase the exposure of the thoracic cavity. A border of muscle should be maintained for reattachment of the diaphragm. Stay sutures or Babcock forceps are used to maintain retraction of the freed portion of the diaphragm and improve visibility. Injury to the nearby hepatic veins and caudal vena cava should be avoided.

Closure

To close the transdiaphragmatic incision, a simple continuous suture line is begun from the most dorsal position of the incision working ventrally and laterally. An absorbable, monofilament suture (eg, 0, 2-0, or 3-0 polydioxanone or similar) is used for closure of the diaphragm. The associated suture needle should be selected with care, with the selection balancing the need for ease of closure with the need to avoid iatrogenic damage to pulmonary or vascular structures. As with the diaphragm incision, care to protect the hepatic veins and caudal vena cava is taken during suturing the diaphragmatic incisions. Once diaphragmatic closure is complete, transdiaphragmatic thoracocentesis is used to restore the subatmospheric pressure differential within the pleural space. Return of the concave appearance of the diaphragm will indicate appropriate evacuation. At this point, abdominal lavage is performed and sponge counts are reconciled. The celiotomy incision is closed in a routine manner.

Thoracostomy Tube Placement

The placement of a thoracostomy (chest) tube after thoracic surgery is not a routine procedure in our practice. This may be a point of controversy for some surgeons, as most retrospective studies have found thoracotomy tubes were placed in greater than 75% of thoracotomy patients.[2,3,30] We make the decision to place a thoracostomy tube based on the expectations of the tube. If there is a significant chance of continued accumulation of air or fluid after surgery, then a chest tube should be placed before recovery. In situations in which the accumulation of fluid or air is thought to be unlikely (eg, PDA ligation or routine lobectomy), then a thoracostomy tube may not be used. Instead, simple thoracocentesis can be performed before anesthesia recovery to remove residual air from the pleural space.

Thoracostomy tubes have been reported to be responsible for several complications after thoracic surgery and unless their presence is medically indicated or they are being used for administration of analgesics or chemotherapeutic agents, they should be removed.[30] Thoracostomy tubes should be removed as soon as they are not performing an essential purpose.

PleuralPorts (Norfolk Vet Products; Skokie, Illinois), a version of a vascular access port, have been used as an alternative to a standard thoracostomy tube. A fenestrated silicon tube is inserted through the thoracic wall into the pleural space. The tubing is connected to a PleuralPort and secured in place. The PleuralPort is then secured to the pericostal tissues and remains in a subcutaneous location. The port is easily palpable through the skin, and after appropriate aseptic preparation of the overlying skin, a Huber needle can be inserted into the port reservoir to aspirate fluid through the port.[31,32]

The advantages of using a PleuralPort after a thoracotomy are that the device can be left in place for an extended period, lack of a need to maintain a thoracic wrap over a chest tube, and the lack of requiring 24-hour patient monitoring. This device is reported to be a good alternative for those patients that will need to have long-term air or fluid removal because of the underlying disease process. We normally place a PleuralPort in dogs undergoing surgery for chylous effusions and have used them for other animals with persistent pleural effusions of neoplastic or idiopathic origins. The primary disadvantages of using a PleuralPort are increased cost compared with a standard chest tube, need to use specialized Huber needles when using the port, and need to eventually remove the port and tubing once there is no further need for fluid removal. So, although the PleuralPort device may not replace a chest tube for the routine postthoracotomy patient, they can be an ideal option for specific-needs patients.

POSTOPERATIVE CARE

Appropriate patient care after thoracic surgery is essential for successful outcomes. Some commonly encountered problems or challenges for the thoracic surgery patient include:

- Incision/wound care: Both lateral thoracostomy and sternotomy procedures have identified wound issues in the postoperative period. Most of these are relatively minor and self-limiting (seromas, hematomas, mild wound dehiscence, or discharge).[2,17–20] Concurrent placements of thoracostomy tubes have resulted in additional wound complications (air leakage and subcutaneous inflammation). Lameness in the ipsilateral foreleg is also reported.[2] This is typically attributed to aggressive extension of the thoracic limbs and the incision of the latissimus dorsi muscle during the standard lateral thoracotomy approach. Preservation of the latissimus muscle and avoiding excessive cranial extension of the foreleg should minimize this problem.[23]
- Analgesia plan: An appropriate analgesia plan is essential for a good outcome after thoracic surgery. The goal of a good analgesia plan should always be to allow the patient to resume normal function as rapidly as possible. Opioid analgesics (eg, fentanyl, morphine, hydromorphone, buprenorphine) should be the mainstay of the analgesia plan.[33] Although the use of constant rate infusions is highly effective, the use of regularly scheduled intermittent analgesic administration can be as effective and is frequently more conducive to nonacademic practices. The historical concern about using opioids after thoracic surgery (ie, respiratory depressant), has been replaced by the knowledge that good analgesia means a more comfortable patient exhibiting more effective respiratory excursions after surgery. Local anesthetic agents (eg, bupivacaine, lidocaine) can be used for local or regional anesthesia (eg, intercostal block,[34] intrapleural anesthesia,[35,36] local

wound anesthesia using an infusion catheter, a splash block, or a lidocaine patch). Other analgesia options include adding nonsteroidal anti-inflammatory drugs, micro doses of α-2 agonists and NMDA agonists (eg, ketamine). A combination of analgesic techniques is routinely used in the postthoracotomy patient.

- Incision management: Daily evaluation of the thoracic wound is appropriate. If a bandage is desirable, a nonadherent dressing is applied over the incision site and secured with a chest wrap. Daily bandage changes are performed until the wound is healed to a point of not needing specific support. If a chest tube is placed, special care needs to be given to the exit site, especially in patients with persistent chylous or inflammatory effusions. Subcutaneous inflammation and secondary infection are possible. Local wound care is essential to minimize problems.

- Respiratory management: For most thoracotomy patients, no special needs are required beyond adequate analgesia. Placement of a nasal oxygen line before the patient recovers from anesthesia can be considered for thoracotomy patients. Preplacing this will allow the stress-free administration of supplement oxygen as required. If there are concerns about continued accumulation of air or fluid within the pleural space, intermittent or continuous evacuation via the thoracostomy tube should be performed. The thoracotomy tubes can be aspirated manually on a regular schedule or on an as-needed basis. If respiratory efforts increase between scheduled aspirations, the patient should be connected to a continuous suction system. If a patient has evidence of pre-existing pulmonary disease or congestion, frequent nebulization and coupage may be beneficial. In addition, postthoracotomy patients are encouraged to get up for a minimal amount of exercise in the immediate recovery period (first 12 hours). In most situations, this may simply mean getting up to go out for elimination needs. If a patient is unable to stand or reposition, a regular schedule for alternating the recumbent side, efforts to keep them in a sternal position, and encouragement to stand should be followed and documented. Nursing support for nutritional and hygienic needs can be critical in nonambulatory patients.

CURRENT CONTROVERSIES/FUTURE CONSIDERATIONS

What is the role of the open thoracotomy in the future? Although there will be a role for minimally invasive surgical (MIS) techniques, the author's opinion is that the lateral thoracotomy and median sternotomy are not going away in the near future. First, the equipment for an open approach is more widely available than is MIS equipment. Furthermore, the cost of MIS equipment for thoracoscopic surgery is significantly more than that of open equipment. The technical skills required for an open procedure is significant but different than the skills needed for effectively evaluating the thoracic cavity with a scope.

SUMMARY

Approaching and closing the thoracic cavity is an achievable procedure for veterinary clinicians; however, success does require careful and honest self-evaluation. Surgical skill and experience, although critically important, are generally not the limiting factor. It is often the availability of trained personnel; adequate facilities for anesthesia, surgery, and postoperative recovery; and critical equipment and ancillary products that create the larger hurdle than surgical skill. Investment in the equipment, training and development of surgical skills and knowledge will allow for the successful introduction of thoracic surgical procedures into the repertoire of a high-quality, general surgery program.

REFERENCES

1. Bellenger CR, Hunt GB, Goldsmid SE, et al. Outcomes of thoracic surgery in dogs and cats. Aust Vet J 1996;74:25–30.
2. Moores AL, Halfacree ZJ, Baines SJ, et al. Indications, outcomes and complications following lateral thoracotomy in dogs and cats. J Small Anim Pract 2007;48: 695–8.
3. Meakin LB, Salonen LK, Baines SJ, et al. Prevalence, outcome and risk factors for post-operative pyothorax in 32 dogs undergoing thoracic surgery. J Small Anim Pract 2013;54:313–7.
4. Robinson R, Chang YM, Seymour CJ, et al. Predictors of outcome in dogs undergoing thoracic surgery (2002-2011). Vet Anaesth Analg 2014;41:259–68.
5. Bigdelian H, Sedighi M. Evaluation of sternal closure with absorbable polydioxanone sutures in children. J Cardiovasc Thorac Res 2014;6:57–9.
6. Orton EC. Thoracic Wall. In: Slatter DA, editor. Textbook of small animal surgery. 3rd edition. Philadelphia: Saunders; 2003. p. 373–87.
7. Hunt GB. Thoracic wall. Chapter 104. In: Tobias KM, Johnston SA, editors. Veterinary surgery: small animal. St. Louis, MO: Elsevier; 2012. p. 1769–86.
8. Radlinsky MG. Thoracic cavity. Chapter 105. In: Tobias KM, Johnston SA, editors. Veterinary surgery: small animal. St. Louis, MO: Elsevier; 2012. p. 1787–812.
9. Monnet E. Lungs. Chapter 103. In: Tobias KM, Johnston SA, editors. Veterinary surgery: small animal. St. Louis, MO: Elsevier; 2012. p. 1752–68.
10. Orton EC, McCracken TO. Small animal thoracic surgery. Philadelphia: William & Wilkens; 1995. p. 55–72.
11. Evans HE. Miller's anatomy of the dog. 3rd edition. Philadelphia: WB Saunders; 1993. p. 290–308.
12. Done SH, Goody PC, Evans SA, et al. Color atlas of veterinary anatomy; the dog & cat, vol. 3. Edinburgh (Scotland): Mosby; 1996. p. 5.1–5.57.
13. Schulman AJ, Lippincott CL. Rib pivot thoracotomy. Compend Contin Educ Pract Vet 1988;10:927–30.
14. Dean PW, Pope ER. Modified intercostal thoracotomy approach. J Am Anim Hosp Assoc 1992;28:87–91.
15. Rooney MB, Mehl M, Monnet E. Intercostal thoracotomy closure: transcostal sutures as a less painful alternative to circumcostal suture placement. Vet Surg 2004;33:209–13.
16. Francel TJ. A rational approach to sternal wound complications. Semin Thorac Cardiovasc Surg 2004;16:81–91.
17. Burton CA, White RN. Review of the technique and complications of median sternotomy in the dog and cat. J Small Anim Pract 1996;37:516–22.
18. Pelsue DH, Monnet E, Gaynor JS, et al. Closure of median sternotomy in dogs: suture vs wire. J Am Anim Hosp Assoc 2002;38:569–76.
19. Ringwald RJ, Birchard SJ. Complications of median sternotomy in the dog and literature review. J Am Anim Hosp Assoc 1989;25:430–4.
20. Williams JM, White RA. Median sternotomy in the dog: an evaluation of the technique in 18 cases [abstract]. Vet Surg 1993;22:246.
21. Chanoit G. Complications after thoracic surgery: don't necessarily blame it on the approach [editorial]. J Small Anim Pract 2013;54:283–4.
22. Losanoff JE, Collier AD, Wagner-Mann CC, et al. Biomechanical comparison of median sternotomy closures. Ann Thorac Surg 2004;71:203–9.
23. Davis KM, Roe SC, Mathews KG, et al. Median sternotomy closure in dogs: a mechanical comparison of technique stability. Vet Surg 2006;35:271–7.

24. Losanoff JE, Foerst JR, Huff H, et al. Biomechanical porcine model of median sternotomy closure. J Surg Res 2002;107:108–12.

25. Nolan TH, Allen HL, Conti PA, et al. Nylon bands for thoracotomy closure. J Am Anim Hosp Assoc 1980;16:759–62.

26. Gines JA, Friend EJ, Vives MA, et al. Mechanical comparison of median sternotomy closure in dogs using polydioxanone and wire sutures. J Small Anim Pract 2011;52:582–6.

27. Luciani N, Anselmi A, Gandolfo F, et al. Polydioxanone sternal sutures for prevention of sternal dehiscence. J Card Surg 2006;21:580–4.

28. Keceligil HT, Kolbakir F, Akar H, et al. Sternal closure with resorbable synthetic loop suture material in children. J Pediatr Surg 2000;35:1309–11.

29. Bright RM, Bright JM, Richardson DR, et al. Clinical and radiographic evaluation of a median sternotomy technique in the dog. Vet Surg 1983;12:13–9.

30. Tattersail JA, Welsh E. Factors influencing the short-term outcome following thoracic surgery in 98 dogs. J Small Anim Pract 2006;47:715–20.

31. Cahalane AK, Flanders JA. Use of pleural access ports for treatment of recurrent pneumothorax in tow dogs. J Am Vet Med Assoc 2012;241:467–71.

32. Cahalane AK, Flanders JA, Steffey MA, et al. Use of vascular access ports with intrathoracic drains for treatment of pleural effusion in three dogs. J Am Vet Med Assoc 2007;230:527–31.

33. Pavlidou K, Papazoglou L, Savvas I, et al. Analgesia for small animal thoracic surgery. Compend Contin Educ Vet 2009;31:432–6.

34. Flecknell PA, Kirk AJ, Liles JH, et al. Post-operative analgesia following thoracotomy in the dog - an evaluation of the effects of bupivacaine intercostal nerve block and nalbuphine on respiratory function. Lab Anim 1991;25:319–24.

35. Conzemius MG, Brockman DJ, King LG, et al. Analgesia in dogs after intercostal thoracotomy: a clinical trial comparing intravenous buprenorphine and intrapleural bupivicaine. Vet Surg 1994;23:291–8.

36. Pascoe PJ, Dyson DH. Analgesia after lateral thoracotomy in dogs-epidural morphine vs intrapleural bupivcaine. Vet Surg 1993;22:144–7.

Current Concepts in Minimally Invasive Surgery of the Abdomen

Milan Milovancev, DVM[a,b,*], Katy L. Townsend, BVSc, MS[a]

KEYWORDS

- Laparoscopy • Dog • Cat • Minimally invasive • Biopsy • Ovariectomy
- Cisterna chyli ablation • Adrenalectomy

KEY POINTS

- Laparoscopic and laparoscopic-assisted procedures are well established in veterinary surgery, with novel minimally invasive approaches and procedures described regularly in the peer-reviewed literature.
- Advances in preoperative work-up (eg, abdominal CT and/or MRI) have facilitated more appropriate patient selection for minimally invasive surgical procedures, allowing more focused dissections and less surgical trauma.
- As the field advances, advantages related to magnification, visualization, and accessibility are expected to establish laparoscopic and laparoscopic-assisted procedures as superior to traditional open surgery for certain procedures.
- Developing advances, such as single-incision laparoscopic surgery (SILS) and/or natural orifice transluminal endosurgery, are actively pursued in veterinary patients.

INTRODUCTION: NATURE OF THE PROBLEM

Minimally invasive surgery of the abdomen is an area of veterinary medicine that continues to progress, paralleling advances in instrumentation, technology, and increasing familiarity of the procedures by newly trained surgeons. Laparoscopic and laparoscopic-assisted procedures are becoming increasingly available to veterinary patients, both in the referral and nonreferral settings, with the American College of Veterinary Surgeons incorporating training in minimally invasive surgery as a required aspect of a residency program. Consequently, many excellent review articles and

---

The authors have nothing to disclose.
[a] Department of Clinical Sciences, College of Veterinary Medicine, Oregon State University, 700 SW 30th Street, Corvallis, OR 97330, USA; [b] Small Animal Surgery, College of Veterinary Medicine, Oregon State University, 267 Magruder Hall, Corvallis, OR 97331, USA
* Corresponding author. Small Animal Surgery, College of Veterinary Medicine, Oregon State University, 267 Magruder Hall, Corvallis, OR 97331.
E-mail address: milan.milovancev@oregonstate.edu

books exist within the veterinary literature, providing detailed equipment descriptions and procedural information related to laparoscopy.[1-5] The purpose of the present article is to supplement these sources by providing readers with an update on more recent developments in the field veterinary laparoscopy and laparoscopic-assisted procedures. Basic equipment setup and procedures are referenced briefly to allow a greater focus on more contemporary procedures and advances in the field.

INDICATIONS/CONTRAINDICATIONS

Indications for laparoscopy include biopsies of almost all organs that can be achieved by laparotomy (**Box 1**). Laparoscopy is also a minimally invasive way to perform several surgical procedures, with more procedures performed as experience and expertise increases (**Box 2**). Ancillary surgical procedures, such as placement of feeding tubes to optimize recovery or to help stabilize patients before procedures, also can be performed (**Box 3**), along with a complete abdominal explore for oncologic staging purposes. Organs and pathology are better seen laparoscopically due to magnification and light source.[5] Targeted biopsies of specific lesions can be performed, obtaining larger samples than could otherwise be achieved percutaneously. Sample procurement via laparoscopy decreases patient morbidity, pain, infection rate, and time compared with a standard laparotomy.[6-9] Other advantages include the ability to document pathology of organs, which is advantageous for developing treatment plans and medical record keeping; monitoring chronic conditions; and education with clients and veterinary colleagues involved in the care of patients.[5]

There are few contraindications to laparoscopy due to the minimally invasive nature of this technique, especially if a traditional laparotomy is warranted. Unstable patients have contraindications for laparoscopy similar to those of laparotomy. Patients with diaphragmatic defects (eg, hernias) should not undergo laparoscopy because insufflated CO_2 expands into the pleural space causing respiratory compromise. Large tumors or mass removals may be best performed with the traditional open approach or surgeries where an obvious conventional surgical approach is warranted. Lack of surgeon experience is a contraindication with laparoscopic procedures, with a steep initial learning curve for this technique. Some surgeons choose to use a predetermined time limit before conversion to traditional methods. Laparoscopy needs specialized surgical equipment, the lack of which is a contraindication.

Box 1
Abdominal organs readily biopsied via laparoscopy

- Liver
- Spleen
- Pancreas
- Lymph nodes
- Kidney
- Adrenal gland
- Peritoneum
- Cholecystocentesis (transhepatic)
- Prostate

Box 2
Established small animal laparoscopic surgical procedures

- Abdominal exploratory
- Ovariectomy, ovariohysterectomy, and/or ovarian remnant removal
- Abdominal cryptorchid testicle removal
- Adrenalectomy
- Cholecystectomy
- Liver lobectomy
- Splenectomy
- Nephrectomy
- CC ablation
- EHPSS attenuation
- Mesenteric lymph node extirpation
- Cystoscopic calculi removal
- Artificial urethral sphincter placement

TECHNIQUE/PROCEDURE
Preparation

Preoperative patient preparation for minimally invasive surgery of the abdomen has many similarities to traditional open abdominal surgery. Preparation includes a routine preoperative fast and use of perioperative antibiotic prophylaxis depending on the planned procedure and patient status. Additional preparation steps include evacuation of the urinary bladder and performing a wider hair clip than might be utilized for a traditional ventral midline laparotomy. Evacuation of the urinary bladder allows for increased physical space within the peritoneal cavity during the laparoscopic procedure as well as minimizing the risk of accidental trauma to the bladder during establishment of laparoscopic portals. A wider hair clip allows for more laterally positioned laparoscopic portal placement to facilitate appropriate instrument triangulation.

Patient Positioning

Patient position for minimally invasive surgery of the abdomen largely depends on the planned procedure. By varying a patient's position, a surgeon can use passive retraction of the abdominal viscera by gravity to facilitate exposure to the anatomic structures of interest for a particular procedure. This position may need to be changed during the procedure, requiring an operating table that can be adjusted to the desired angles. For procedures involving the retroperitoneal space, it is often advantageous to

---

Box 3
Laparoscopic tube placement options

- Gastrostomy tube
- Jejunostomy tube
- Cystostomy tube
- Cholecystostomy tube

position patients in sternal recumbency, with the pelvis supported, allowing abdominal viscera to passively fall away from retroperitoneal structures of interest.[10]

An ideal operating table for use with minimally invasive surgery allows tilting the table side to side (eg, to provide sequential access to each side of the reproductive tract) as well as the front and back ends of the table (eg, Trendelenburg position to maximize exposure to the caudal abdomen). It is important to carefully secure patients to the table to prevent inadvertent slipping or falling during the procedure. Commercially available tabletop add-on patient positioning platforms are becoming more common through veterinary laparoscopic supply companies. These devices offer the ability to retrofit an existing nontilting surgical table for laparoscopic use.

Approach

The surgical approach for minimally invasive surgery of the abdomen varies depending on the planned procedure. Even for a single specific procedure, the number of planned portals may vary depending on surgeon preference, which may dictate changes in the specific port placement. In general, many laparoscopic procedures use portals along the ventral aspect of the abdomen in a baseball field configuration to help with triangulation of instruments. Alternative approaches for specific procedures to facilitate exposure for particular organs are, however, important to consider. For example, a paralumbar approach may be used for adrenalectomy and greatly facilitates exposure of the gland during the procedure.[10] Use of a 0° telescope inserted into a screw-in threaded trocar as it is being established is useful for direct identification of tissues/organ the port is advancing toward.

Technique/Procedure

Basic technical and equipment-related information is available in excellent review articles, both previously published in this series as well as in other sources.[1–5] This review emphasizes modern port options and instruments necessary for some of the newer and evolving minimally invasive surgical procedures performed in the abdominal cavity.

Laparoscopic instruments portals have evolved beyond the traditional Veress needle and/or Hasson methods. Portals that accommodate variable instruments sizes are commercially available (**Fig. 1**) and greatly facilitate swapping of instruments and telescopes of different sizes during a procedure. Optical trocars that allow direct visualization of tissues as they are penetrated during portal placement are helpful, especially

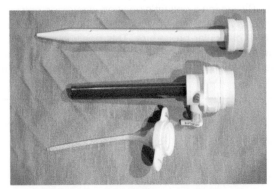

Fig. 1. A laparoscopic portal that automatically accommodates and seals around instruments or telescopes ranging from 5 mm to 12 mm in diameter.

when placing a portal through a nontraditional location (eg, paracostal portal placement for an adrenalectomy). Portals that warm, clean, and defog the telescope during insertion are available as well. Finally, simple blunt-tip screw-in trocars (**Fig. 2**) allow for safer entry into the abdomen without creation of a larger body wall defect or a need for retention sutures as required with the traditional Hasson technique. Wound retraction devices for laparoscopic-assisted procedures are available to facilitate exposure through a relatively small surgical incision.[11]

As more advanced and diverse laparoscopic procedures are described for small animal veterinary patients, the selection of instruments that are necessary is also increasing. For example, laparoscopic cotton-tipped dissectors (**Fig. 3**) and both 5-mm and 10-mm laparoscopic right-angled forceps (**Fig. 4**) are invaluable for dissection of adrenal tumors and gall bladders. New tip options for the LigaSure vessel sealing device (Covidien, Mansfield, Massachusetts) have facilitated dissection of tissues using the same instrument notably faster and easier (eg, Dolphin tip and/or Maryland jaw instruments).

A summary of laparoscopic and laparoscopic-assisted procedures is provided.

Liver biopsy

Indications for a liver biopsy include unexplained laboratory or abnormal imaging findings. Diagnosing liver dysfunction is normally achieved by histopathology, ensuring that liver biopsy is a common procedure performed. The liver is a simple and easily accessible organ to be laparoscopically biopsied.[3,5,12] A coagulation panel should be considered before biopsy. Generally, a 2-port position is used: ventral midline for the camera and either a right or left cranial quadrant paramedian instrument portal. Both sides of the liver can be biopsied through either side. A 5-mm × 10-mm oval cup biopsy forceps is the easiest way, obtaining a sample from the edge of the lobe or from the central liver parenchyma. The tissue is grasped gently and held for 10 to 30 seconds before it is either gently tugged or twisted away. The biopsy area should be visualized until the bleeding has ceased. If bleeding is prolonged, pressure can be applied to the biopsy site with a cotton-tipped applicator or a piece of gelatin sponge, or oxidized regenerated cellulose can be placed over the biopsy site. A third port can be placed on the contralateral side to use either a coagulation device or a pretied loop

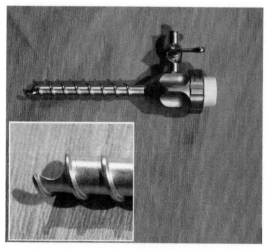

Fig. 2. A blunt-tip screw-in trocar. Inset shows a close-up view of the tip.

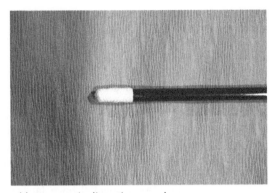

Fig. 3. Cotton-tipped laparoscopic dissecting wand.

ligature or extracorporeally assembled loop ligature in patients with coagulopathy. Multiple sites should be biopsied from multiple lobes for best chance of diagnostic accuracy.

Cholecystocentesis
Aspiration of bile for culture and analysis is often needed when assessing hepatopathies. An 18G or 20G long needle with an inner stylet (eg, cerebrospinal fluid collection needle) is used. The needle should enter caudal to the last rib to prevent puncture of the diaphragm and pneumothorax. The gall bladder should be punctured by first advancing the needle through the quadrate lobe of the liver, so, if leakage occurs, it drains back into the liver. Often, abdominal insufflation pressures need to be reduced to allow the needle to reach the gall bladder.

Pancreatic biopsy
Indications for pancreatic biopsy include differentiation of acute pancreatitis versus acute liver disease and visualization of both organs.[13,14] The tip of the right limb of the pancreas is usually the most accessible area. The pancreas needs to be visualized to determine if this is a representative sample; however, the left limb of the pancreas is challenging to assess completely.[5] A 5-mm × 10-mm oval biopsy cup forceps can be used on the periphery to ensure that the pancreatic ducts and the blood supply to pancreas and the duodenum are not compromised. Either a ventral or right lateral laparoscopic approach can be used. Laparoscopic-assisted biopsy of the pancreas can be

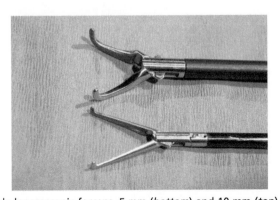

Fig. 4. Right-angle laparoscopic forceps, 5 mm (*bottom*) and 10 mm (*top*).

used by externalizing the descending duodenum through an incision for gastrointestinal biopsies. Other methods include a pretied loop, a LigaSure device, harmonic scalpel, and hemostatic clips.[5] Pancreatitis as a complication of pancreatic biopsy is low.[15]

Spleen biopsy and splenectomy

There are few indications for splenic biopsy, with the procedure generally performed to assess for neoplasia.[16] Diffuse splenomegaly is generally the indication, instead of splenic masses; 5-mm × 10-mm oval cup biopsy forceps are used. A coagulation profile should be performed before biopsy. A ventral or left lateral midabdominal approach should be used. If splenomegaly is suspected, caution should be taken when entering the abdomen with either approach. Coagulation through the use of a piece of gelatin sponge or oxidized regenerated cellulose can be placed over the biopsy site.

Laparoscopic splenectomy has been reported using a 3-port technique with patients in dorsal recumbency and rolled into right lateral recumbency or with a SILS Port (Covidien, Mansfield, Massachusetts).[17,18] A vessel sealant device is used to perform a hilar splenectomy. A specimen retrieval bag should be used to prevent seeding of the abdomen, and incisions may need to be enlarged to the remove the spleen.

Lymph node extirpation

Detection of an enlarged lymph node during laparoscopy or by imaging is an indication for biopsy, along with nondiagnostic cytology aspirates, and during staging of canine oncologic patients. Three-mm or 5-mm oval cup biopsy forceps are used, and patient positioning depends on other laparoscopic procedures performed concurrently or on which node is sampled.

Laparoscopic medial iliac lymph node (MILN) extirpation has been reported.[19] Indications include diagnostic staging of canine oncologic patients. A lateral 3-portal caudal abdominal approach can be used for the ipsilateral lymph nodes. MILNs are identified by incising the retroperitoneum caudal to the deep circumflex iliac artery and vein and dorsal to the external artery or vein using a vessel sealant device. This technique was successful in 8 purpose-bred hounds with normal MILNs. The contralateral MILN was not able to be seen or biopsied from this approach. Also, the hypogastric and sacral lymph nodes cannot be visualized or sampled. Complications include hemorrhage and tearing of lymph node capsule. Further work is necessary before this technique becomes a routinely clinically feasible option.

Kidney biopsy and nephrectomy

Kidney biopsies are generally obtained only when they change the course of treatment. Examples of such scenarios may include the need to obtain a specific diagnosis, define the extent of disease, and determine the reversibility of renal disease. Laparoscopic-assisted biopsies are obtained with a needle core biopsy instrument (14G or 16G) under visualization.[3,5] Osmotic diuretics that improve renal blood flow should be discontinued before biopsy, and a coagulation profile should be assessed. Port placement can be ventral midline with patients rotated slightly, with the kidney to be biopsied up or in a midabdominal location away from the falciform fat on midline. The needle core biopsy instrument should enter near the kidney, relatively high on the lateral body wall. The angle of the needle needs to be tangential to the kidney to obtain a cortical biopsy, and the throw of the needle biopsy instrument needs to be considered to avoid injury to surrounding structures. After the biopsy is taken, the tip of a palpation probe or cotton-tipped applicator should be placed over the biopsy site for 1 minute.[3] The major complication of kidney biopsy is hemorrhage, and patients likely have hematuria for the next 24 to 48 hours. Fluid diuresis should be used postbiopsy to prevent blood clot formation and obstruction.[5]

Laparoscopic left nephrectomy has been described in an experimental series of 16 dogs.[20] Dogs were placed in dorsal recumbency in a 15° Trendelenburg position and a 3-port technique used. The animals were then rolled onto the right side to start the dissection. The renal vessels were be ligated with ligating clips and sectioned. The kidney were freed from the peritoneum and the ureter was mobilized. The ureter was ligated and divided at the level of the iliac vessels. The kidney was removed with a specimen retrieval bag and needed to be morselized. This technique has also been performed in a clinical series of 9 dogs.[21] This method differed by early dissection of the ureter which aids in retraction and elevation of the kidney for dissection and division of the ureter near its insertion into the bladder instead of near the iliac vessels. Complications include visual obstruction due to hydroureter and hemorrhage. Conversion to an open approach may be necessary.

Laparoscopic-assisted gastrointestinal biopsies
Biopsies of the small intestine can be performed in a laparoscopic-assisted manner.[22] The animal is placed in dorsal recumbency and standard midline portals are established. The jejunum can be atraumatically grasped and exteriorized through an enlarged portal incision. Standard intestinal samples then can be obtained. Wound retraction devices can be used to aid in larger segments of intestinal exteriorization, also allowing the duodenum and ileum to be sampled more easily.

Laparoscopic ovariectomy, ovariohysterectomy, or ovarian remnant removal
Laparoscopic ovariectomy or ovariohysterectomy is a common procedure and one many veterinary surgeons begin their laparoscopic career with. Advantages over a traditional open approach include enhanced visualization and faster recovery.[9] Patients are placed in dorsal recumbency, on a table that has the ability to tilt to the left and right; 1-, 2-, and 3-port techniques have all been described. The 1-port technique relies on having an operating scope, consisting of a 10-mm operating scope with an operating channel that accommodates 5-mm instruments. A common technique is a 2-port technique, where a subumbilical port is placed, and second port is placed either cranial or caudal to the subumbilical port. Patients are rotated into right or left lateral recumbency, opposite to the side of ovariectomy, and the ovary is identified. It is then held up to the body wall and suspended to the body wall by a percutaneous swaged-on needle with suture or laparoscopic hook. A vessel sealant device may be used to remove the ovary. If the ovary is suspended by a suture, the ovary can remain in place and be removed after the contralateral ovariectomy, or it may be removed immediately if a laparoscopic hook is used. A 3-port technique can be used where all 3 ports are placed in midline, with 2 caudal to the umbilicus and 1 cranial to the umbilicus.[23] This method does not involve suspending the ovary from the abdominal wall.

The 3-port technique can be used to perform an ovariohysterectomy.[5] Bilaterally, the ovarian pedicles are transected and the broad ligament is also transected close to the uterus to decrease number of blood vessels as well as to minimize potential damage to the ureters and gastrointestinal tract with the electrosurgical device. This is performed from cranial to caudal, with constant traction on the proper ligament. The ovaries and uterus are exteriorized through the caudal incision, where the body of the uterus is ligated and transected in a routine manner. Complications include hemorrhage and other standard laparoscopic complications.

Ovariohysterectomy for pyometra also can be performed using the 3-port technique.[24] A wound retractor device can be used in the caudal portal to facilitate removal of the uterus. Careful case selection is warranted, with guidelines suggested for dogs less than 10 kg with a uterine horn diameter less than 2 cm, or dogs greater than 10 kg with a uterine horn diameter less than 4 cm. Potential complications include uterine rupture and hemorrhage. The authors have performed laparoscopic ovarian remnant removals using both 2- and 3-port techniques.

Laparoscopic cryptorchid testicle removal

The laparoscopic cryptorchid testicle removal procedure is indicated after identification of an abdominally located testis.[22,25] Patients should be placed in Trendelenburg position and can be rolled into left and right lateral recumbency depending on location of testicle. A subumbilical port is placed and the retained testicle is found. A 2-port technique can be used by placing the second port over the testicle and using Babcock forceps or an aggressive grasper to elevate the testicle outside the body wall after extending the second port incision and ligating the vasculature and vas deferens routinely.[25] Alternatively, a 3-port technique can be used to ligate the vasculature intra-abdominally, with either a vessel sealant device or hemoclips.[5] The portal site still needs to be enlarged to remove the testicle.

Laparoscopic adrenalectomy

Laparoscopic adrenalectomy has been described in canine patients.[3,10,26] Appropriate case selection is paramount to success due to the pertinent anatomy of the gland near large vascular structures and an adrenal gland tumor's ability to invade these structures. Imaging of adrenal masses is important preoperatively, with vessel invasion a contraindication for laparoscopic removal along with large size (>6 cm). Unstable patients should have an open approach. The standard work-up for an adrenal mass should be performed as per open adrenalectomy, along with appropriate medications before surgery is performed. Dogs can be placed either in lateral recumbency with elevation of the erector spinae muscle group or in sternal recumbency with 2 cushions placed to elevate the chest and the pelvic area to leave the abdomen unsupported.[10,26] A 3- or 4-port technique should be used, in the paralumbar fossa, caudal to the last rib on a virtual half circle triangulating the approximate position of the adrenal gland. A fourth port can be used dorsally for retraction if needed. The laparoscope may be placed in the middle port, with instruments on either side, or at either the cranial or caudal ports, depending on individual anatomy. For exposure, the kidneys need to be retracted caudally or dorsally and, for right adrenalectomy, the right lateral hepatic lobe needs to retracted cranially. After exposure of the adrenal gland and dissection through the peritoneum dorsolateral to the gland, the phrenicoabdominal vein should be ligated. A combination of a vessel sealant device, bipolar electrocautery, and dissecting forceps should be used to circumferentially dissect the gland. Careful dissection is needed to ensure that the capsule stays intact. Once the gland is dissected free, the adrenal gland and tumor can be placed in a specimen retrieval bag and removed. Potential complications include lost visualization during minor bleeding or lymphatic vessel damage, profuse bleeding requiring immediate conversion to an open approach, and rupture of the adrenal gland and mass.

Laparoscopic cisterna chyli ablation

The laparoscopic cisterna chyli (CC) ablation procedure is indicated as an adjunct procedure for idiopathic chylothorax treatment. CC ablation may reduce backpressure in the thoracic duct and may reduce the force driving recanalization. Dogs are placed in sternal recumbency with the pelvis elevated. This technique can be performed with 2 portals placed 2- to 3-cm caudal to the 13th rib on the left side in the dorsal third of the abdomen, or with a transdiaphragmatic portals placed in the dorsal third of the left 10th or 11th intercostal space (use of nonvalved port is critical to prevent tension pneumothorax).[27] Initial dissection is through the craniolateral aspect of the peritoneum between the lateral margin of the left kidney and the dorsolateral body wall. The renal artery is identified and followed to the aorta. The CC is located dorsal to the aorta in the region of the left renal artery. The sternal positioning allows the kidney to displace ventrally during dissection. To facilitate identification of the CC, the popliteal lymph node is injected with methylene blue. The ablation is performed by blunt tearing of the wall of the CC. Complications include inability to locate the CC, tension pneumothorax, and diaphragmatic tears in the transdiaphragmatic approach and aortic laceration. Only surgeons experienced with laparoscopy should attempt this procedure.

Laparoscopic cholecystectomy

Indications for laparoscopic cholecystectomy are uncomplicated gall bladder mucoceles.[3,28] Complicated mucoceles, such as cases of coagulopathies, bile peritonitis, extrahepatic biliary tract obstruction, and small body size (<4 kg), are contraindications, along with surgeon inexperience. Patients should be placed in dorsal recumbency and a 4-port technique is generally used: a subumbilical port, a left cranial quadrant port, and 2 right cranial quadrant ports, triangulated around the anticipated position of the gall bladder. A Trendelenburg position should be adopted. A fan retractor should be placed in the left port, the laparoscope in the right-sided port closest to midline and the other right port along with the subumbilical port for instruments controlled by the surgeon. The cystic duct needs to be dissected round, proximal to the first hepatic duct. The duct is then ligated either with hemoclips or suture and then the gall bladder is dissected off the hepatic fossa. If any leakage of bile occurs or hemorrhage, an open approach should be performed. The gall bladder should be placed in a specimen retrieval bag for removal. Complications include cystic duct rupture, potential for confusion between the cystic and common bile duct, and bile spillage from the cystic duct ligation. Recommendations are to double ligate the cystic duct with monofilament suture by extracorporeal or intracorporeal knots. A liver biopsy for bacterial culture and histopathology along with a bile culture should be performed.

Laparoscopic extrahepatic portosystemic shunt ligation

Laparoscopic extrahepatic portosystemic shunt (EHPSS) ligation is indicated for patients with a single congenital EHPSS.[5,29] Patients are placed in dorsal recumbency, on a table that is able to be tilted head up and from left to right. A 4-portal ventral abdominal technique is used: 1 portal caudal to the umbilicus, left and right paramedian (also called midabdominal by some investigators) portals, and a portal in the right caudal quadrant equidistant from the umbilicus and pubic bone. Gastric traction sutures should be used to aid in elevation of the stomach for identification of the shunt. The animal can be rotated into left lateral recumbency to aid the visualization of the epiploic foramen by elevating the descending duodenum. The animal can be rotated into right lateral recumbency to assess the left abdominal gutter and the diaphragm, to assess for portoazygous or portophrenic shunts. The omental bursa can be assessed with patients in dorsal recumbency. Once the vessel is identified, it is dissected out and cellophane with ligating clips is placed. The pancreas and the jejunum should be visualized to assess for signs of portal hypertension.

Laparoscopic-assisted cystoscopic calculus removal

Urinary calculi can be removed through laparoscopic-assisted cystoscopy.[30–33] Patients should be placed in the Trendelenburg position. The camera portal should be placed 2- to 3-cm caudal to the umbilicus, with a second site caudally on midline for female patients and paramedian or midline for male patients. The apex of the bladder is grasped with Babcock forceps through the caudal port and used to retract the bladder to the abdominal wall where a ventral cystotomy can be made just large enough to allow removal of the largest cystolith. The bladder is temporarily sutured to the abdominal wall and a cystocope or laparoscope can be used to visualize the bladder lumen, remove cytsoliths, and take biopsies for histopathology or culture. Alternatively, the cystoliths can be removed by flushing saline into the bladder at 300 mm Hg and removed via suction after temporary cystopexy to avoid urine contamination into the abdominal cavity. The proximal urethra should be evaluated for remnant uroliths. The bladder wall then can be closed primarily.

Gastropexy

Prophylactic gastropexy can be performed either laparoscopically or with a laparoscopic-assisted procedure, with pexy tensile strengths comparable to open gastropexy methods and ultrasonographically documented intact gastropexies at more than 1 year postoperatively.[34,35] With the laparoscopic procedure, the creation of the pexy is performed either via intracorporeal suturing or with laparoscopic stapling devices.[36,37] A modified laparoscopic technique has been described in experimental dogs using extracorporeal percutaneous full-thickness body wall sutures to hold a cauterized gastric serosa against a cauterized peritoneal surface.[38] Most recently, laparoscopic gastropexy has been described using single-port access with articulating instruments and angled telescopes.[39] Laparoscopic-assisted gastropexy is favored by some surgeons because it is technically simpler to perform and does not require specialized equipment beyond a basic laparoscopic set up.[34,37]

Feeding and/or drainage tubes

Laparoscopic and laparoscopic-assisted feeding and drainage tube placement has been described in experimental and clinical dogs. Laparoscopic-assisted enterostomy tube placement is an effective method for feeding tube placement in a minimally invasive manner.[40,41] Laparoscopic cystostomy tube placement, along with cystopexy, has been described using a 3-portal technique.[42] Temporary biliary drainage can be established via laparoscopic-guided percutaneous cholecystostomy tube placement using a locking-loop pigtail catheter and has been shown superior to ultrasound-guided techniques in a cadaver study.[43]

COMPLICATIONS AND MANAGEMENT

Potential complications of minimally invasive surgery of the abdomen depend on the specific procedure performed. Generally speaking, the types of complications that can be encountered are similar to those associated with traditional open surgical procedures (**Box 4**), with a few differences discussed later.

Complications specific to laparoscopic procedures early in a surgeon's career may arise from a lack of appropriate exposure or visualization, inappropriately rough tissue handling exacerbated by the lack of tactile feedback with long laparoscopic instruments, or general inexperience with the advanced procedures performed. For these reasons, it is important that a surgeon beginning laparoscopy seek appropriate training and guidance and progress in a stepwise fashion from simpler procedures and/or laparoscopic-assisted procedures to more advanced delicate procedures near critical anatomic structures. Electing to convert to an open approach to prioritize patient health and safety should not be viewed as a failure.

Other laparoscopic-specific complications are related to the generation of capnoperitoneum, often associated with excessive intra-abdominal pressures. Such pressures can cause impaired venous return to the heart and/or compression of the diaphragm with subsequent respiratory compromise. To avoid these issues, many

> **Box 4**
> **Complications associated with minimally invasive surgery of the abdomen**
>
> - Hemorrhage
> - Seroma
> - Accidental penetration of an abdominal organ during portal placement
> - Wound dehiscence
> - Insufflation-related complications
>   - Acid-base disturbances
>   - Reduced venous return to the heart
>   - Impaired diaphragmatic movement and reduced pulmonary function
> - Procedure-specific complications (feeding or draining tube leakage, tumor seeding at portal locations, etc.)

surgeons prefer to use low intra-abdominal insufflation pressures (6–10 cm H_2O), with only brief periods of higher pressure as needed to perform specific brief maneuvers (eg, provide counterpressure against the force required to establish additional portals). At the completion of a laparoscopic procedure, the peritoneal cavity should be completely deflated to remove CO_2 gas.

POSTOPERATIVE CARE

- Monitoring
  - Baseline temperature, pulse, and respiration on completion of the procedure and every 6–8 hours thereafter
  - If concern for hemorrhage, packed cell volume/total solids and regular arterial blood pressure monitoring
  - Depending on patient status, consider monitoring electrolytes, acid-base status, specific organ parameters (eg, renal panel), corticotropin stimulation test postadrenalectomy, urination frequency and volumes, and respiratory status.
- Analgesics
  - Opioids (hydromorphone, fentanyl, buprenorphine, etc.)
    - Dose and frequency dictated by extent of the procedure and regular patient pain score assessment
  - If no contraindications, consider adding a nonsteroidal anti-inflammatory drug
    - May be used in combination with opioids
    - For less-invasive procedures, may be used alone or after a brief period of opioid analgesia
  - Local incisional blocks can reduce need for systemic analgesics
    - For example, bupivicaine at portal sites
- Supportive care
  - Nutritional support is an important consideration
    - If not eating well on own, consider feeding tube placement during anesthetic episode associated with the surgery
  - Maintain hydration status, typically with intravenous crystalloid and/or colloid fluids
    - Avoid overhydration
  - Prevent self-trauma (eg, via use of Elizabethan collars, as needed); restrict activity

REPORTING, FOLLOW-UP, AND CLINICAL IMPLICATIONS

Results from clinicopathologic samples and tests obtained during an abdominal minimally invasive procedure dictate the long-term follow-up plans and clinical implications. Referral to board-certified specialists may be indicated (eg, internal medicine specialist for a chronic hepatopathy documented via laparoscopic liver biopsy or medical oncologist for an adrenal cortical adenocarcinoma removed via laparoscopy). Other follow-up is best performed with a primary care veterinarian (eg, long-term dietary modification as dictated by urolith analysis results obtained during a laparoscopic-assisted cystoscopy).

OUTCOMES

Patient recovery after minimally invasive surgical procedures of the abdomen typically is rapid and, therefore, long-term outcomes usually depend on the underlying disease process rather than the surgery itself. Elective procedures, such as gastropexy and/or gonadectomy, are expected to yield excellent long-term outcomes. Conversely, biopsy results indicating a disseminated neoplastic process carry a worse prognosis; minimally invasive surgical procedures often can yield critical long-term prognostic information while sparing patients the increased morbidity associated with a traditional open procedure.

CURRENT CONTROVERSIES/FUTURE CONSIDERATIONS

SILS is becoming increasingly popular to reduce complications and surgical trauma of multiple sites. This technique can be achieved through a specialized operating telescope that has a working channel; however, only 1 instrument can be used at a time. The SILS Port is a multiple instrument port that allows the telescope, insufflation, and 2 instrument portals. The difficulty in using this instrument can arise from the inability to appropriately triangulate instruments. Articulating instruments are available that decrease the collision of instruments. SILS has been described in ovariectomy, gastropexy, splenectomy, and laparoscopic-assisted intestinal surgery.[18,23,39,44]

Lift laparoscopy is a feasible alternative to traditional capnoperitoneum laparoscopy and has been used in clinical dogs undergoing ovariohysterectomy.[45–47] A custom-made elliptical lift device is inserted into the peritoneal cavity via a ventral midline stab incision and traction is applied to provide a working space for the desired laparoscopic procedure. Lift location and number of lift devices (eg, 2 lift devices applied simultaneously with 1 in a more cranial location and the other placed caudally) may provide better access to different portions of the peritoneal cavity. This alternative method of providing physical space within the peritoneal cavity for laparoscopic procedures may be beneficial in a subset of critically ill patients who might not tolerate the potential physiologic alterations associated with capnoperitoneum.[45]

Natural orifice transluminal endoscopic surgery is an emerging technique that enables surgery to be performed on abdominal organs by access through the stomach, colon, or vagina. Ovariectomy via the stomach has been reported in research and clinical dogs.[48]

SUMMARY

Minimally invasive surgery of the abdomen continues to be an advancing field within the discipline of veterinary surgery. Many traditional procedures can now be performed in a minimally invasive manner, allowing for quicker patient recovery and less associated tissue trauma. Biopsies of most abdominal organs are readily performed in a minimally invasive manner. As veterinary surgeons become more familiar with laparoscopy, advanced procedures are becoming increasingly commonplace. Certain laparoscopic procedures are expected to replace their corresponding traditional open surgeries.

REFERENCES

1. Lansdowne JL, Mehler SJ, Boure LP. Minimally invasive abdominal and thoracic surgery: techniques. Compend Contin Educ Vet 2012;34(5):E2.
2. Lansdowne JL, Mehler SJ, Boure LP. Minimally invasive abdominal and thoracic surgery: principles and instrumentation. Compend Contin Educ Vet 2012;34(5):E1.
3. Mayhew PD. Advanced laparoscopic procedures (hepatobiliary, endocrine) in dogs and cats. Vet Clin North Am Small Anim Pract 2009;39(5):925–39.
4. Monnet E, Twedt DC. Laparoscopy. Vet Clin North Am Small Anim Pract 2003; 33(5):1147–63.
5. Rawlings CA. Laparoscopy. In: Tams TR, Rawlings CA, editors. Small animal endoscopy. 3rd edition. St Louis (MO): Elsevier; 2011. p. 397–477.
6. Hancock RB, Lanz OI, Waldron DR, et al. Comparison of postoperative pain after ovariohysterectomy by harmonic scalpel-assisted laparoscopy compared with median celiotomy and ligation in dogs. Vet Surg 2005;34(3):273–82.
7. Davidson EB, Moll HD, Payton ME. Comparison of laparoscopic ovariohysterectomy and ovariohysterectomy in dogs. Vet Surg 2004;33(1):62–9.
8. Devitt CM, Cox RE, Hailey JJ. Duration, complications, stress, and pain of open ovariohysterectomy versus a simple method of laparoscopic-assisted ovariohysterectomy in dogs. J Am Vet Med Assoc 2005;227(6):921–7.
9. Culp WT, Mayhew PD, Brown DC. The effect of laparoscopic versus open ovariectomy on postsurgical activity in small dogs. Vet Surg 2009;38(7): 811–7.
10. Naan EC, Kirpensteijn J, Dupre GP, et al. Innovative approach to laparoscopic adrenalectomy for treatment of unilateral adrenal gland tumors in dogs. Vet Surg 2013;42(6):710–5.
11. Gower SB, Mayhew PD. A wound retraction device for laparoscopic-assisted intestinal surgery in dogs and cats. Vet Surg 2011;40(4):485–8.
12. Petre SL, McClaran JK, Bergman PJ, et al. Safety and efficacy of laparoscopic hepatic biopsy in dogs: 80 cases (2004-2009). J Am Vet Med Assoc 2012; 240(2):181–5.
13. Webb CB, Trott C. Laparoscopic diagnosis of pancreatic disease in dogs and cats. J Vet Intern Med 2008;22(6):1263–6.
14. Barnes RF, Greenfield CL, Schaeffer DJ, et al. Comparison of biopsy samples obtained using standard endoscopic instruments and the harmonic scalpel during laparoscopic and laparoscopic-assisted surgery in normal dogs. Vet Surg 2006;35(3):243–51.
15. Harmoinen J, Saari S, Rinkinen M, et al. Evaluation of pancreatic forceps biopsy by laparoscopy in healthy beagles. Vet Ther 2002;3(1):31–6.
16. Radhakrishnan A, Mayhew PD. Laparoscopic splenic biopsy in dogs and cats: 15 cases (2006-2008). J Am Anim Hosp Assoc 2013;49(1):41–5.
17. Collard F, Nadeau ME, Carmel EN. Laparoscopic splenectomy for treatment of splenic hemangiosarcoma in a dog. Vet Surg 2010;39(7):870–2.
18. Khalaj A, Bakhtiari J, Niasari-Naslaji A. Comparison between single and three portal laparoscopic splenectomy in dogs. BMC Vet Res 2012;8:161.

19. Steffey MA, Daniel L, Mayhew PD, et al. Laparoscopic extirpation of the medial iliac lymph nodes in normal dogs. Vet Surg 2014. http://dx.doi.org/10.1111/j. 1532-950X.2014.12207.x.

20. Kim YK, Park SJ, Lee SY, et al. Laparoscopic nephrectomy in dogs: an initial experience of 16 experimental procedures. Vet J 2013;198(2):513–7.

21. Mayhew PD, Mehler SJ, Mayhew KN, et al. Experimental and clinical evaluation of transperitoneal laparoscopic ureteronephrectomy in dogs. Vet Surg 2013;42(5): 565–71.

22. Mayhew P. Surgical views: techniques for laparoscopic and laparoscopic assisted biopsy of abdominal organs. Compend Contin Educ Vet 2009;31(4): 170–6.

23. Case JB, Marvel SJ, Boscan P, et al. Surgical time and severity of postoperative pain in dogs undergoing laparoscopic ovariectomy with one, two, or three instrument cannulas. J Am Vet Med Assoc 2011;239(2):203–8.

24. Adamovich-Rippe KN, Mayhew PD, Runge JJ, et al. Evaluation of laparoscopic-assisted ovariohysterectomy for treatment of canine pyometra. Vet Surg 2013; 42(5):572–8.

25. Miller NA, Van Lue SJ, Rawlings CA. Use of laparoscopic-assisted cryptorchidectomy in dogs and cats. J Am Vet Med Assoc 2004;224(6):875–8, 865.

26. Jimenez Pelaez M, Bouvy BM, Dupre GP. Laparoscopic adrenalectomy for treatment of unilateral adrenocortical carcinomas: technique, complications, and results in seven dogs. Vet Surg 2008;37(5):444–53.

27. Sakals S, Schmiedt CW, Radlinsky MG. Comparison and description of transdiaphragmatic and abdominal minimally invasive cisterna chyli ablation in dogs. Vet Surg 2011;40(7):795–801.

28. Mayhew PD, Mehler SJ, Radhakrishnan A. Laparoscopic cholecystectomy for management of uncomplicated gall bladder mucocele in six dogs. Vet Surg 2008;37(7):625–30.

29. Miller JM, Fowler JD. Laparoscopic portosystemic shunt attenuation in two dogs. J Am Anim Hosp Assoc 2006;42(2):160–4.

30. Arulpragasam SP, Case JB, Ellison GW. Evaluation of costs and time required for laparoscopic-assisted versus open cystotomy for urinary cystolith removal in dogs: 43 cases (2009-2012). J Am Vet Med Assoc 2013;243(5):703–8.

31. Pinel CB, Monnet E, Reems MR. Laparoscopic-assisted cystotomy for urolith removal in dogs and cats - 23 cases. Can Vet J 2013;54(1):36–41.

32. Rawlings CA, Mahaffey MB, Barsanti JA, et al. Use of laparoscopic-assisted cystoscopy for removal of urinary calculi in dogs. J Am Vet Med Assoc 2003; 222(6):759–61, 737.

33. Runge JJ, Berent AC, Mayhew PD, et al. Transvesicular percutaneous cystolithotomy for the retrieval of cystic and urethral calculi in dogs and cats: 27 cases (2006-2008). J Am Vet Med Assoc 2011;239(3):344–9.

34. Rivier P, Furneaux R, Viguier E. Combined laparoscopic ovariectomy and laparoscopic-assisted gastropexy in dogs susceptible to gastric dilatation-volvulus. Can Vet J 2011;52(1):62–6.

35. Wilson ER, Henderson RA, Montgomery RD, et al. A comparison of laparoscopic and belt-loop gastropexy in dogs. Vet Surg 1996;25(3):221–7.

36. Hardie RJ, Flanders JA, Schmidt P, et al. Biomechanical and histological evaluation of a laparoscopic stapled gastropexy technique in dogs. Vet Surg 1996; 25(2):127–33.

37. Rawlings CA. Laparoscopic-assisted gastropexy. J Am Anim Hosp Assoc 2002; 38(1):15–9.

38. Mathon DH, Dossin O, Palierne S, et al. A laparoscopic-sutured gastropexy technique in dogs: mechanical and functional evaluation. Vet Surg 2009;38(8): 967–74.

39. Runge JJ, Mayhew PD. Evaluation of single port access gastropexy and ovariectomy using articulating instruments and angled telescopes in dogs. Vet Surg 2013;42(7):807–13.

40. Rawlings CA, Howerth EW, Bement S, et al. Laparoscopic-assisted enterostomy tube placement and full-thickness biopsy of the jejunum with serosal patching in dogs. Am J Vet Res 2002;63(9):1313–9.

41. Hewitt SA, Brisson BA, Sinclair MD, et al. Evaluation of laparoscopic-assisted placement of jejunostomy feeding tubes in dogs. J Am Vet Med Assoc 2004; 225(1):65–71.

42. Zhang JT. Laparoscopy for percutaneous tube cystostomy in dogs. J Am Vet Med Assoc 2010;236(9):975–7.

43. Murphy SM, Rodriguez JD, McAnulty JF. Minimally invasive cholecystostomy in the dog: evaluation of placement techniques and use in extrahepatic biliary obstruction. Vet Surg 2007;36(7):675–83.

44. Manassero M, Leperlier D, Vallefuoco R, et al. Laparoscopic ovariectomy in dogs using a single-port multiple-access device. Vet Rec 2012;171(3):69.

45. Fransson BA, Grubb TL, Perez TE, et al. Cardiorespiratory changes and pain response of lift laparoscopy compared to capnoperitoneum laparoscopy in dogs. Vet Surg 2014. http://dx.doi.org/10.1111/j.1532-950X.2014.12198.x.

46. Kennedy KC, Fransson BA, Gay JM, et al. Comparison of pneumoperitoneum volumes in lift laparoscopy with variable lift locations and tensile forces. Vet Surg 2014. http://dx.doi.org/10.1111/j.1532-950X.2014.12306.

47. Fransson BA, Ragle CA. Lift laparoscopy in dogs and cats: 12 cases (2008-2009). J Am Vet Med Assoc 2011;239(12):1574–9.

48. Freeman L, Rahmani EY, Burgess RC, et al. Evaluation of the learning curve for natural orifice transluminal endoscopic surgery: bilateral ovariectomy in dogs. Vet Surg 2011;40(2):140–50.

Current Concepts in Minimally Invasive Surgery of the Thorax

MaryAnn Radlinsky, DVM, MS

KEYWORDS

- Thoracic • Endoscopic • Surgery • Thoracoscopy

KEY POINTS

- Thoracoscopic surgery is a rapidly expanding field of surgery that can greatly decrease patient morbidity.
- Thoracoscopic surgery provides magnification and lighting to improve the ability to visualize structures in the chest.
- Thoracoscopy can be used for many procedures commonly performed via open surgery.

INTRODUCTION

Thoracoscopy is a rapidly advancing field of surgical intervention in dogs and cats. Its clinical use was first described in 1998,[1] and since that time many advances have been made. The differences in patient recovery, compared with open thoracic surgery, have been shown and make sense because the trauma of the approach is greatly reduced.[1] The approaches classically used with open surgery can be mimicked with thoracoscopy; however, the use of thoracoscopy should not be seen as an alternative to open thoracotomy. Complications with thoracoscopy require the surgeon to convert to thoracotomy, and the equipment and skill for those approaches and surgical means of addressing complications must be available in an instant.[2] The standard thoracotomy is via an intercostal or median sternotomy, and thoracoscopy can be done with the same approaches, maintaining the anatomy in a normal view with which the surgeon is familiar. Changes in position or viewing angle can offer new views, such as those seen when the patient is placed in sternal recumbency or when operating the left ligamentum for correction of esophageal constriction associated with persistent right aortic arch from a caudal direction.[3,4] This article introduces thoracoscopy to practitioners to make the procedure more familiar as an option for minimally invasive diagnostic and therapeutic interventions.

Disclosures: The author has nothing to disclose.

Small Animal Medicine and Surgery, College of Veterinary Medicine, The University of Georgia, DW Brooks Drive, Athens, GA 30602-7390, USA

E-mail address: radlinsk@uga.edu

INDICATIONS/CONTRAINDICATIONS

The indications for thoracoscopy are the same as those for open thoracotomy and include thoracic exploration for pleural effusion, chronic pulmonary disease, pericardial effusion, pyothorax, division of the ligamentum arteriosum, and chylothorax. Clinicians performing thoracoscopy should be capable of and prepared for conversion to open thoracotomy, including having the appropriate equipment in the operative suite.

Contraindications for thoracoscopy include concurrent conditions that increase the risk associated with general anesthesia or are problematic with open surgery. Other contraindications include significant adhesions that limit the ability to progress with thoracoscopy and very large lesions that require open thoracotomy for retrieval.[5]

ANESTHESIA

As with open thoracic procedures, anesthesia must be tailored to the ventilatory needs of the patient and positive ventilation is required because of the loss of negative pleural pressure on creation of a pneumothorax. Standard withholding of food should be observed, and the premedication equal to that of open thoracotomy. As with open thoracic procedures, local anesthetic can be added to the regimen and is easily done around each port site. Monitoring equipment should be as rigidly used as it is with open thoracotomy and should include electrocardiogram, pulse oximetry (oxygen saturation), capnography (end-tidal carbon dioxide [CO_2] measurement), and blood pressure measurement. Many surgeons prefer direct rather than indirect blood pressure measurement with thoracic procedures because the ability to obtain blood gas measurements is achieved with an arterial catheter. Arterial blood gas measurement may be required to tailor ventilatory needs for any type of thoracic surgery. In addition to ventilation, positive end-expiratory pressure may be required if specialized ventilation is done (eg, 1-lung ventilation [OLV]).[6]

OLV is not usually required for thoracoscopy. Simply creating a pneumothorax and altering the means of ventilation usually creates enough working space for thoracoscopy. OLV is achieved by the use of specialized endotracheal tubes that have 1 tube extending down and into 1 bronchus with another opening in the trachea. This type of tube allows anesthetists to selectively ventilate right or left sides, depending on the tube connected to the ventilator (BronchoPart, Rusch Inc, Teleflex Medical, Research Triangle Park, NC). A simpler means of providing OLV is to use a long, narrow endotracheal tube selectively into 1 bronchus or to block 1 bronchus with a balloon-tipped catheter (Arndt Endobronchial Blocker, Cook Medical, Bloomington, IN). Regardless of the method chosen, OLV should be established in the operative suite to ensure proper maintenance of the desired lung, and requires flexible endoscopic guidance for selective bronchial intubation or bronchial blockage with a balloon; however, blind placement may be possible and confirmed with thoracoscopic appearance of atelectasis.[7] Loss of OLV is problematic in the reported studies on completely thoracoscopic pneumolobectomy, the only procedure for which OLV is required.[8,9]

The most common starting point for altering ventilation during thoracoscopy without OLV is to decrease the tidal volume by half and increase the ventilator rate 2-fold. Monitoring equipment is extremely important, because each patient does not respond equally to this change in ventilation and more adjustments may be needed to optimize CO_2 and oxygen levels. Alterations noted in animals in most experimental studies are within survivable limits; however, the studies were done on normal animals.[10,11] Decreased Pao_2 and increased $Paco_2$ are to be expected.[10,11] These changes are caused by increased ventilation perfusion (V/Q) mismatch caused by shunting. The changes were likely minimized in reported research because of hypoxemic vasocon-striction in the normal animals studies; normal lungs undergo vasoconstriction of poorly oxygenated segments.[10,11] This response may or may not be maintained in patients undergoing thoracoscopy for diseased states.

EQUIPMENT
Imaging Equipment

The equipment needed for thoracoscopy is significant in amount and cost and is main-tained on a mobile tower or on a boom in a dedicated surgical suite. The endoscope is of first and foremost importance. Zero and 30°rigid endoscopes are commonly used in veterinary surgery, but the 30° endoscope is required for thoracoscopy to allow viewing of the entire thorax or hemithorax without undue pressure and leverage against the ribs (**Fig. 1**).[12] Levering against the rib can cause patient discomfort and puts the fragile endoscope at risk of damage.[12] The endoscope and projection system provide great magnification, which is one of the benefits of endoscopic surgery beyond the decreased morbidity related to a minimally invasive approach. Endo-scopes are also described by their outer diameter, with the 5-mm endoscope being most versatile for small animal practice; however, 10-mm and 2.7-mm diameters are also available for larger and smaller dogs and cats.

A camera is attached to the endoscope and is largely responsible for the image quality obtained. Cameras are available in entry-level to high-definition qualities. A strong light source is required to provide one of the great advantages of endoscopic surgery: lighting at the target. A xenon light source is best for viewing the thoracic cavity.[12] The light source is connected to the endoscope via a light guide cable; care must be taken to avoid damage to it, which diminishes the quality of the light entering the endoscope. The image should be viewed on a high-quality monitor capable of matching a medical-grade monitor. Image capture is also usually desired for documentation and client education. Current image processors can record to compact disc (CD), digital versatile disc (DVD), and universal serial bus (USB). Because procedures are done within the rigid thorax, insufflation is not required, unlike laparoscopy, in which CO_2 must be infused into the peritoneal space to separate the body wall from the viscera. Some experts use very low levels of CO_2 infusion during the most complex procedures and for feline thoracoscopy; however, this can compli-cate anesthesia and is not recommended for average surgeons.[13,14] Thus, a CO_2 cannister and insufflator are not standard for thoracoscopy.

Ports

Access into the thoracic cavity for instruments and the endoscope must maintain the desired minimal trauma to the thoracic wall. Repeated instrument passages could

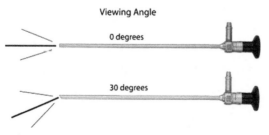

Viewing Angle

0 degrees

30 degrees

Fig. 1. The difference between the 0° (*top*) and 30° (*bottom*) endoscope. The 30° endoscope allows for viewing within the rigid confines of the chest without levering against the ribs.

result in damage to the skin, subcutis, muscle, or most importantly the neurovascular bundles. Ports protect the soft tissues from such damage and come in many shapes, sizes, and materials. Metal or plastic ports are available; the latter may be rigid or flexible. Rigid ports may be smooth or threaded, with threaded ports becoming more popular because of their ability to maintain position despite multiple instrument changes, which are required for more advanced procedures (**Fig. 2**). Flexible ports can be maintained in position by suturing their cuff to the skin and may be more desirable because they do not compress neurovascular bundles against the ribs (**Fig. 3**).

Specialized Devices

Specialized instrumentation is typically used for thoracoscopic procedures, although thoracoscopic-assisted procedures have been described using more traditional instrumentation.[15,16] Instrumentation must be narrow enough to enter the thorax through the port; must function on the end of a long shaft; and usually have interchangeable types of handles that ratchet, can ratchet, or do not ratchet (appropriate for scissors) (**Fig. 4**). Other specialized devices must be deliverable through the narrow ports and include retractors, specimen retrieval bags, or ligating loops. These specialized instruments must be capable of expanding once inside the chest cavity.

Most interventional thoracoscopy is done with the aid of energy devices, such as attaching monopolar electrocautery to instruments, using the harmonic scalpel, or by use of a vessel-sealing device. Energy devices can be vital to simple (eg, pericardectomy) or advanced procedures to minimize the need for conversion to open surgery. Pretied loop ligatures may be useful for controlling hemorrhage or sampling (eg, lung). Specialized staplers can be used in the thorax (endoscopic gastrointestinal anastomosis [GIA; Covidien, Mansfield, MA] stapler or endoscopic clip applier [Multi-Fire 10 mm Clip Applier, Microline Surgical, Beverly, MA]) or thoracoscopic-assisted

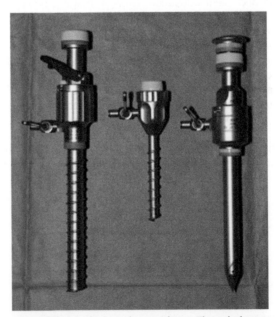

Fig. 2. Rigid ports are available with threads or without. Threaded ports are often used for paraxiphoid access to the thoracic cavity with the patient in dorsal recumbency.

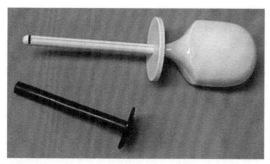

Fig. 3. Smooth, flexible ports are valuable for intercostal placement because they avoid compression of the neurovascular bundles against the ribs.

procedures can use standard stapling devices such as the thoracoabdominal (TA; Covidien, Mansfield, MA) stapler outside the thorax.

THORACOSCOPIC APPROACHES

The type of approach used to evaluate the thorax depends on the desired outcome because a lateral approach allows full examination of 1 hemithorax and a paraxiphoid approach mimics the median sternotomy and allows examination of both hemithoraces but not the most dorsal aspects of the chest cavity. Port placement may be blind, under endoscopic guidance, or via a minithoracotomy. Blind placement is not recommended, because it requires a sharp trocar to pass the port through the thoracic wall and puts intrathoracic structures at risk. Endoscopic guidance can be achieved after the first port is in place, and subsequent ports can be placed with either sharp or blunt trocars. Sharp incision of the skin is followed by passing the port on its trocar into the chest. A miniapproach can be used with any type of trocar; a small incision is made through the skin and blunt dissection is used before port insertion. Threaded ports may or may not have a trocar, depending on their tips. Threads help to maintain the port's position during the procedure.

Lateral thoracoscopy is done with the patient in right or left lateral recumbency and the approach mimics and should allow the standard open thoracotomy to be done if needed in case of emergency. Ports should be placed in the intercostal spaces that allow access to the desired target organ. Many different port sites have been described for division of the ligamentum arteriosum for persistent right aortic arch (PRAA), thoracic duct ligation, partial or complete pneumolobectomy, mediastinal

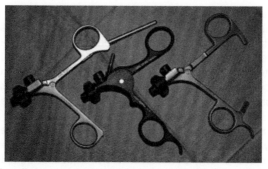

Fig. 4. Ratcheted handles or nonratcheting handles available for endoscopic instruments.

mass removal, lymph node biopsy, and pleural biopsy. Ports should be placed via a minithoracotomy or under endoscopic visualization after the first port is in place. Pushing on the external intercostal space with a finger or instrument while visualizing the site with the endoscope inside the chest can help to ensure that the port will allow access to the desired structure once in place; the desired target should be visualized adjacent to the port site or at a distance from it, depending on the access required. Ports should not be too close to the target or the scope, but should allow visual entry of instruments by the endoscope before advancing them to the target structure. More distant port placement is required for instruments with a long working end, such as the endoscopic GIA stapler, because placing the port too close to the targeted hilus hinders opening of the jaws of the instrument if it is still inside the port when it reaches the site. Thought should be put into the need for a retractor in cases in which the target is close to the lung (PRAA).

A paraxiphoid approach may be needed for exploration of both hemithoraces for diseases of unknown cause (eg, undiagnosed pleural effusion) or for ventral procedures (eg, pericardectomy). This approach mimics the median sternotomy, which is required if conversion to open surgery becomes necessary. A threaded port (Ternamian EndoTIP, Karl Storz, Goleta, CA) is generally the port of choice for this type of approach. The port is placed by slowly advancing it into the chest adjacent to the base of the xiphoid process. The port traverses the diaphragm and should be directed at a modest ventral angle (approximately 30°) into the ipsilateral hemithorax. Visual advancement through the diaphragm and into the chest is possible and is greatly desired to ensure that the port does not simply enter the mediastinum. A 0° endoscope is required with a commercially available stopper that maintains the endoscope's position in the port to avoid the endoscope exiting the port and contacting the tissues, leading to loss of visualization. Once the paraxiphoid port is in place, the ipsilateral thorax can be examined. Division of the mediastinum is required for entry into and examination of the contralateral thorax. Doing so requires an instrument port placed intercostally to permit insertion of a grasper and scissors or vessel-sealing device to free the mediastinum from the sternum. Intercostal ports should be ventral enough to avoid the pulmonary excursions during ventilation, minimizing the risk of inadvertent damage during instrument passages.

PROCEDURES
Diagnostic Procedures

Diagnostic procedures include sampling of the pleura, mediastinum, pericardium, lung, and lymph nodes. Each is done with cup biopsy forceps on exposure of the appropriate tissue or with a pretied loop, which is required for lung biopsy.

Pleural and mediastinal biopsy

The pleura is easily sampled with 5-mm cup biopsy forceps; however, damage to the intercostal vasculature can be fatal, so care should be taken to avoid it.[5] If the intercostal vessels are not visible, attention to the anatomy is essential. The intercostal vessels are situated along the caudal aspect of each rib. Palpation of the intercostal space and associated rib is used to guide placement of the biopsy forceps in the center of the intercostal space and avoid the rib at the cranial aspect of the chosen intercostal space. As with all endoscopic biopsy techniques, the site is observed after sampling to ensure that no significant hemorrhage is present. The mediastinum is sampled similarly, but visual avoidance of the vasculature must be done to direct the site to be sampled. Energy devices are rarely needed for sampling the pleura or mediastinum.

Pericardial biopsy

The pericardium can be sampled with grasping forceps to elevate it away from the epicardium and Metzenbaum-type scissors are used to remove a sample. Visualization and avoidance of the vessels are usually simple with thoracoscopy. Confirmation of minimal hemorrhage is required, as it is for pleural and mediastinal sampling. Pericardectomy (or pericardial window) should be considered unless only a small piece of pericardium is desired. If the pericardium is sufficiently thick and well vascularized, consider using an energy device during sampling; monopolar cautery can be attached to Metzenbaum scissors or a vessel-sealing device can be used.

Lung biopsy

Peripheral lung biopsy can be done by applying a pretied loop ligature to the lung for diffuse pulmonary disease. Approximately 2 cm of lung can be sampled with this technique.[17] A pretied loop ligature is placed in the chest adjacent to the target, and grasping forceps pass through the loop and elevate the tip of lung, which is ligated by tightening the loop (**Fig. 5**). The tip of lung is transected with scissors, and the suture end severed with hook scissors. Use of a vessel-sealing device has been described in experimental study, but its clinical use has not been defined and requires investigation before it can be recommended.[18] The lung must be evaluated for hemorrhage and air leakage after sampling.

Lymph node biopsy

Lymph nodes may be sampled thoracoscopically and should be evaluated histopathologically in every case of pulmonary neoplasia. They are located adjacent to important vascular structures, and, along with pneumolobectomy, lymph node sampling is considered an advanced technique. The mediastinum should be carefully elevated before removal or biopsy. A 5-mm cup biopsy forceps can be used for sampling; alternatively, the lymph node can be dissected and removed. Energy devices may be necessary for lymph node biopsy. Tracheobronchial lymph node anatomy has been mapped recently, and OLV was described for the procedure to identify and remove them.[19] Difficulties with OLV, hemorrhage, and ability to locate the lymph nodes were reported.[19]

Interventional Procedures

Interventional procedures include pericardectomy, mass removal, mediastinal debridement for pyothorax, division of the ligamentum arteriosum for PRAA, partial

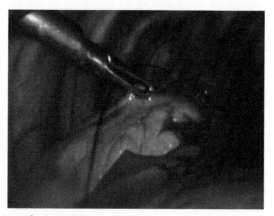

Fig. 5. The periphery of a lung lobe is encircled with a pretied loop ligature and grasped with Babcock forceps for sampling.

or complete pneumolobectomy, and thoracic duct ligation. Nearly all of the interventional procedures use specialized instrumentation such as a vessel sealer or stapling device.

Pericardectomy/pericardial window

Thoracoscopic pericardectomy was one of the earliest and most accepted procedures adopted from human surgery.[1] The procedure can be done in lateral or dorsal recumbency; the dorsally recumbent procedure is most common. After a paraxiphoid port is in place, 2 more ports are required to retract the pericardium and incise it.[20] The 2 instrument ports can be on the same side of the chest, but most often 1 is placed in a caudal intercostal space (8th to 10th) on each side of the chest. The pericardium is elevated away from the epicardium, and a window created ventrally. Energy is usually used by connecting monopolar cautery to the Metzenbaum-type scissors or more commonly by using a vessel-sealing device. A pericardial window may be adequate for treating pericardial effusion associated with neoplasia, but it is not adequate for long-term survival for idiopathic pericardial effusion.[20] Once the pericardial window has been made, filleting the pericardium with 3 incisions from the window extending to 1 cm ventral to the phrenic nerves allows an open pericardium that should not allow herniation and entrapment of part of the heart.[3] A subtotal pericardectomy can be achieved with the patient in dorsal recumbency; the pericardium ventral to the phrenic nerves is removed, taking care to avoid phrenic nerve trauma directly or via thermal spread. Alternating OLV may provide an increased visual space to decrease the risk of phrenic nerve damage, but it does not eliminate the risk.[21] Cases of effusion related to right auricular masses may be treated completely thoracoscopically with mass excision and pericardectomy if masses are amenable to stapling.[22]

Mediastinal mass removal

Mediastinal mass removal may require OLV and has been described for noninvasive thymomas.[23] Mass resection used a harmonic scalpel on lesions of 4.5 cm or less.[23] The procedure is done in dorsal recumbency with ports in the paraxiphoid and caudal and midthoracic intercostal spaces on either the same or opposite sides of the thorax, and, as with other mass removals, use of a specimen retrieval bag is recommended.

Mediastinal debridement

Mediastinal debridement for pyothorax is an extension of the skills necessary for mediastinal sampling and pericardectomy. The anatomy must be strictly protected, including the internal thoracic artery and vein, phrenic nerves, heart, and diaphragm. Dorsal recumbency is necessary for removal of the ventral mediastinum and perhaps for pericardectomy if the pericardium is involved. Energy is usually required, and initial exploration should be done to ensure that the mass of mediastinum is not so large as to require immediate median sternotomy and to ensure that significant adhesions are not present so as to increase the risk of organ trauma or unduly increase surgery time. Samples should be preserved for histopathologic evaluation and aerobic, anaerobic, and fungal culture. If foreign material has been identified on preoperative diagnostic testing, it must be removed.

Persistent right aortic arch

PRAA can be treated with thoracoscopy; however, the diagnosis of PRAA and not another vascular ring anomaly should be made before the start of surgery. The patient is placed in right lateral recumbency and ports are placed to view and operate the ligamentum arteriosum from a ventral or caudal angle.[4,24] Three instrument ports are usually required: 2 for grasping and dissecting and 1 for pulmonary retraction of the left cranial lung lobe. Ports placed at the third, fifth, and seventh intercostal spaces for instruments and the endoscope in a triangulated fashion can be augmented with a second port in the seventh intercostal space for lung retraction.[4] Alternatively, all ports may be placed in the sixth or seventh intercostal space for dissection from caudal to cranial, thus affecting only 1 intercostal space and simplifying application of local anesthestic.[25] The ligamentum must be identified caudal to the dilated esophagus and once completely dissected it is either clipped with an endoscopic clip applier or sealed before division (**Fig. 6**). The magnification and lighting of thoracoscopy greatly enhance the ability to remove remaining fibers from the esophagus.

Pneumolobectomy

Partial or complete pneumolobectomy can be achieved completely thoracoscopically or with thoracoscopic assistance.[26] The endoscope is used to locate the abnormal segment of lung, which is often a mass lesion or emphysema, bullae, or blebs associated with pneumothorax.[9,27,28] With assisted partial or complete pneumolobectomy, the abnormal segment of lung is identified and exteriorized (**Fig. 7**). One port site must be extended; use of an Alexis wound retractor is ideal because it opens the site and protects it from metastasis, trauma, and perhaps infection.[26,29] A standard TA stapler can be used for the procedure once the lung is exteriorized.[25,26] The average surgery time was approximately 90 minutes, and no intraoperative complications were reported.[26] The associated hilar lymph nodes must be examined and sampled in cases of pulmonary neoplasia. Completely endoscopic pneumolobectomy requires the use of an endoscopic GIA stapler and 3 to 4 ports.[8,9] This device is large and long, and an appropriate port must be placed distant from the hilus to allow the jaws to open unhindered by the port (**Fig. 8**). The dorsally located pulmonary ligament must be divided for caudal lung lobectomy. The stapler is positioned across the hilus of the lung to be removed; indicator lines on the stapler help the surgeon ensure that the entire hilus is stapled. Firing of the device places 6 rows of staples across the hilus and divides between them centrally. The lung should be placed in a specimen retrieval bag for removal through a port site, which must be enlarged enough for passage of the bag. Port site enlargement for either the assisted or completely endoscopic procedure should not include retraction that would tear the musculature or rib articulations with

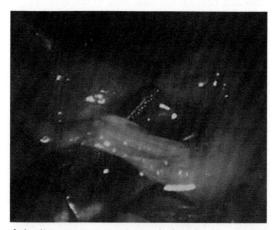

Fig. 6. Dissection of the ligamentum arteriosum before ligation and division for thoracoscopic treatment of PRAA.

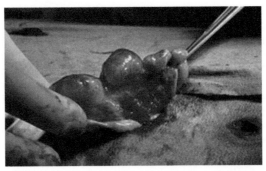

Fig. 7. Lung exteriorized via extension of 1 intercostal port. The segment of lung can be resected using an assisted technique with standard stapling equipment.

the spine or sternum, otherwise the minimal invasiveness of the procedure is lost. Conversion to an open approach occurred in 9% of the dogs in the most recent report of pneumolobectomy and was done for reasons typically including failure to maintain OLV, poor visualization, or a large mass.[8]

Thoracic duct ligation

Thoracic duct ligation can be done in sternal or lateral recumbency. En masse ligation of all structures dorsal to the aorta can be done caudal to the entry of the azygous vein and ventral to the sympathetic trunks.[3,30] Either en masse ligation or individual ligation with endoscopic clips may be done for ductal occlusion. Coloration is not required for en masse ligation but is useful following ligation to ensure that no patent branches remain.[3,30] The duct may be visualized before or following ligation with methylene blue infusion 0.25 to 0.5 mg/kg via a popliteal lymph node, injection of a mesenteric lymph node, by catheterization of an intestinal lymphatic, or by injection of the diaphragmatic crus.[31] Large volumes may be reliably infused after partial exposure of the convex surface of the lymph node. The distal pole should be stabilized and a butterfly catheter needle inserted into the medulla of the lymph node for gradual, gentle infusion of dye. The author commonly performs laparoscopic cisterna chyli ablation following thoracic duct ligation, and then turns the patient into dorsal recumbency for pericardial window and fillet for the treatment of chylothorax.[3]

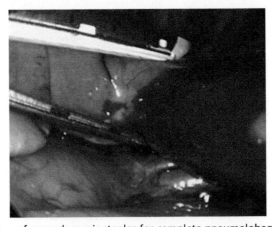

Fig. 8. Introduction of an endoscopic stapler for complete pneumolobectomy.

AFTERCARE

Once intrathoracic procedures are complete, most of the ports should be removed and endoscopically evaluated to ensure that intercostal vessel damage has not occurred. A thoracostomy tube should be placed to evacuate the chest and to monitor for postoperative pneumothorax or hemorrhage. The tube should be placed through its own site and not through a previous port site to avoid air entry into the chest around the tube. Thoracoscopy can be used to view thoracostomy tube placement and to verify that the tube is ideal in its position. All port sites should be closed in 3 layers: muscle, subcutis, and skin. Port sites should be treated with local anesthetic if not already done. Patients should be placed in the intensive care unit, as they would be for open surgery, and should be monitored for dyspnea, pneumothorax, hemorrhage, and proper oxygenation. Nasal oxygen or an oxygen cage can be used until the patient's atelectasis has clinically resolved. The thoracostomy tube should be maintained for a duration equal to that used for the same type of surgery done in standard open fashion. Analgesia should be accomplished and tailored to the patient's needs.

COMPLICATIONS AND MANAGEMENT

As mentioned earlier, surgeons should be capable and should have all of the necessary equipment in the operative suite for immediate conversion to open thoracotomy for any complication associated with the surgery or with thoracoscopy. Complications associated with thoracoscopy in particular include pulmonary or mediastinal hemorrhage, which can occur if instruments are passed without endoscopic visualization.[2] Special care should be taken to avoid sampling over obvious vessels, and, if not visible, the pleura should be sampled in the middle or caudal aspect of the intercostal space, which should remain palpable despite pleural thickening. Extreme care should be taken when dissecting and sampling tracheobronchial lymph nodes, because of the large vessels adjacent to the lymph nodes. Hemorrhage may be addressed with endoscopic clips, loop ligatures, intracorporeal knot tying for ligation, or with an energy device. Access and visualization are important, and evacuation of hemorrhage with suction is helpful. Blood transfusion and reoperation may be required to treat hemorrhage and should be pursued as for open surgery, which may be required instead of thoracoscopy for complications.

Pneumothorax is another serious complication and may require reoperation; however, continuous suction may allow minor pulmonary trauma to heal without surgery. Avoidance of pneumothorax can be achieved by maintaining a wide view and visual confirmation of lack of trauma during instrument introduction; the view can be made narrow once all instruments have reached the target site. One-lung ventilation may be necessary for pneumolobectomy, but is not usually used to decrease pulmonary trauma, because of its consequences with ventilation. The lungs should be evaluated on completion of surgery before closure of the port sites to ensure lack of air leakage. If leaks are identified, they should be treated with partial pneumolobectomy using a stapling device, pretied loop ligature, or via complete pneumolobectomy.[2]

Conversion to open surgery may be done during thoracoscopy if ventilation cannot be made adequate to meet the oxygenation and ventilatory needs of the patient, or if significant pulmonary trauma or hemorrhage is seen during the procedure. Conversion may also be done if the surgery time is significantly long or if adhesions are present that interfere with surgical progression.

FUTURE DIRECTIONS

As equipment and technology improve, more progress is expected in thoracoscopy in veterinary patients. More advanced procedures include pericardioscopy and right atrial appendage mass removal.[22,31] Complete extirpation of tracheobronchial lymph nodes improves the staging of cancer in canine patients, and has been described using thoracoscopy.[19] Future research is likely to focus on specialized imaging for neoplasia to improve complete excision and mapping of lymph nodes for staging.

SUMMARY

Thoracoscopy is a technique that can greatly reduce patient morbidity associated with thoracic procedures. The reduced trauma of the approach and dramatic magnification and lighting are attractive for some procedures (eg, thoracic duct ligation). However, thoracoscopy does not obviate intercostal thoracotomy or median sternotomy, because these open techniques are required for complications during or after thoracoscopy and for large masses or when widespread adhesions are present. Significant accumulation of fat in the thorax is a relative contraindication for thoracoscopy, because it limits visualization of structures. Thoracoscopic surgery is becoming more widespread and more techniques are being developed, increasing the ability of veterinary surgeons to minimize patient discomfort following significant internal surgery.

REFERENCES

1. Walsh PJ, Remedios AM, Ferguson JF, et al. Thoracoscopic versus open partial pericardectomy in dogs: comparison of postoperative pain and morbidity. Vet Surg 1999;28:472–9.
2. Radlinsky MG. Complications and need for conversion from thoracoscopy to thoracotomy in small animals. Vet Clin North Am Small Anim Pract 2009;39: 977–84.
3. Allman DA, Radlinsky MG, Ralph AG, et al. Thoracoscopic thoracic duct ligation and thoracoscopic pericardectomy for treatment of chylothorax in dogs. Vet Surg 2010;39:21–7.
4. MacPhail CM, Monnet E, Twedt DC. Thoracoscopic correction of persistent right aortic arch in a dog. J Am Anim Hosp Assoc 2001;37:577–81.
5. Schmiedt C. Small animal exploratory thoracoscopy. Vet Clin North Am Small Anim Pract 2009;39:953–64.
6. Kudnig ST, Monnet E, Riquelme M, et al. Effect of positive end-expiratory pressure on oxygen delivery during 1-lung ventilation for thoracoscopy in normal dogs. Vet Surg 2006;35:534–42.
7. Mayhew PD, Culp WT, Pascoe PJ, et al. Evaluation of blind thoracoscopic-assisted placement of three double-lumen endobronchial tube designs for one-lung ventilation in dogs. Vet Surg 2012;41:664–70.
8. Mayhew PD, Hunt GB, Steffey MA, et al. Evaluation of short-term outcome after lung lobectomy for resection of primary lung tumors via video-assisted thoracoscopic surgery or open thoracotomy in medium- to large-breed dogs. J Am Vet Med Assoc 2013;243:681–8.
9. Lansdowne JL, Monnet E, Twedt DC, et al. Thoracoscopic lung lobectomy for treatment of lung tumors in dogs. Vet Surg 2005;34:530–5.
10. Kudnig ST, Monnet E, Riquelme M, et al. Cardiopulmonary effects of thoracoscopy in anesthetized normal dogs. Vet Anaesth Analg 2004;31:121–8.

11. Faunt KK, Cohn LA, Jones BD, et al. Cardiopulmonary effects of bilateral hemi-thorax ventilation and diagnostic thoracoscopy in dogs. Am J Vet Res 1998;59: 1494–8.

12. Van Lue SJ, Van Lue AP. Equipment and instrumentation in veterinary endoscopy. Vet Clin North Am Small Anim Pract 2009;39:817–37.

13. Daly CM, Swalec-Tobias K, Tobias AH, et al. Cardiopulmonary effects of intratho-racic insufflation in dogs. J Am Anim Hosp Assoc 2002;38:515–20.

14. Polis I, Gasthuys F, Gielen I, et al. The effects of intrathoracic pressure during continuous two-lung ventilation for thoracoscopy on the cardiorespiratory param-eters in sevoflurane anaesthetized dogs. J Vet Med A Physiol Pathol Clin Med 2002;49:113–20.

15. Borenstein N, Behr L, Chetboul V, et al. Minimally invasive patent ductus arterio-sus occlusion in 5 dogs. Vet Surg 2004;33:309–13.

16. Laksito MA, Chambers BA, Yates GD. Thoracoscopic-assisted lung lobectomy in the dog: report of two cases. Aust Vet J 2010;88:263–7.

17. Adamiak Z, Holak P, Piórek A. Thoracoscopic biopsy of lung tumors using a Roeder's loop in dogs. Pol J Vet Sci 2008;11(1):75–7.

18. Mayhew PD, Culp WT, Pascoe PJ, et al. Use of the Ligasure vessel-sealing device for thoracoscopic peripheral lung biopsy in healthy dogs. Vet Surg 2012;41:523–8.

19. Steffey MA, Daniel L, Mayhew PD, et al. Video-assisted thoracoscopic extirpation of the tracheobronchial lymph nodes in dogs. Vet Surg 2014. [Epub ahead of print].

20. Case JB, Maxwell M, Aman A, et al. Outcome evaluation of a thoracoscopic peri-cardial window procedure or subtotal pericardectomy via thoracotomy for the treatment of pericardial effusion in dogs. J Am Vet Med Assoc 2013;242:493–8.

21. Mayhew KN, Mayhew PD, Sorrell-Raschi L, et al. Thoracoscopic subphrenic peri-cardectomy using double-lumen endobronchial intubation for alternating one-lung ventilation. Vet Surg 2009;38:961–6.

22. Ployart S, Libermann S, Doran I, et al. Thoracoscopic resection of right auricular masses in dogs: 9 cases (2003-2011). J Am Vet Med Assoc 2013;242:237–41.

23. Mayhew PD, Friedberg JS. Video-assisted thoracoscopic resection of noninva-sive thymomas using one-lung ventilation in two dogs. Vet Surg 2008;37:756–62.

24. Isakow K, Fowler D, Walsh P. Video-assisted thoracoscopic division of the liga-mentum arteriosum in two dogs with persistent right aortic arch. J Am Vet Med Assoc 2000;217:1333–6.

25. Monnet E. Interventional thoracoscopy in small animals. Vet Clin North Am Small Anim Pract 2009;39:965–75.

26. Wormser C, Singhal S, Holt DE, et al. Thoracoscopic-assisted pulmonary surgery for partial and complete lung lobectomy in dogs and cats: 11 cases (2008-2013). J Am Vet Med Assoc 2014;245:1036–41.

27. Brissot HN, Dupre GP, Bouvy BM, et al. Thoracoscopic treatment of bullous emphysema in 3 dogs. Vet Surg 2003;32:524–9.

28. Case JB, Mayhew PD, Singh A. Evaluation of video-assisted thoracic surgery for treatment of spontaneous pneumothorax and pulmonary bullae in dogs. Vet Surg 2014. [Epub ahead of print].

29. Brisson BA, Reggeti F, Bienzle D. Portal site metastasis of invasive mesothelioma after diagnostic thoracoscopy in a dog. J Am Vet Med Assoc 2006;229:980–3.

30. Radlinsky MG, Mason DE, Biller DS, et al. Thoracoscopic visualization and liga-tion of the thoracic duct in dogs. Vet Surg 2002;31:138–46.

31. Bayer BJ, Dujowich M, Krebs AI, et al. Injection of the diaphragmatic crus with methylene blue for coloration of the canine thoracic duct. Vet Surg 2014;43: 829–33.

Current Concepts in Wound Management and Wound Healing Products

Jacqueline R. Davidson, DVM, MS

KEYWORDS

- Wound management • Wound products • Moist wound healing • Bandaging
- Autolytic debridement

KEY POINTS

- Autolytic debridement is a type of selective debridement in which the body's own immune system removes unhealthy tissue and contaminants.
- The contact layer of the bandage can be used to maintain a moist wound environment, which can promote autolytic debridement and wound healing.
- Selection of the most appropriate contact layer is based on the stage of wound healing and the amount of exudate being produced.

INTRODUCTION

Open wounds must often be managed for days to weeks until they can be closed or they heal by second intention. Most wounds will heal without complications. Basic wound care incorporates the principles of aseptic technique and gentle tissue handling. In addition, many wound care products are available that will potentially debride the wound without damaging healthy tissue, reduce infection, and improve the rate of wound healing. This article is an overview of some of the current wound dressings, topical products, and modalities used in the management of open wounds.

INITIAL MANAGEMENT

Care of traumatic wounds may begin immediately after wounding by covering the wound with a clean, dry bandage to prevent further contamination and reduce hemorrhage (**Box 1**). A bandage also stabilizes the tissues to reduce further trauma and improve comfort. Potentially life-threatening conditions should be addressed before performing detailed wound management. Thorough wound assessment may require

The author has nothing to disclose.
Veterinary Small Animal Clinical Sciences, College of Veterinary Medicine & Biomedical Sciences, Texas A&M University, 4474 TAMU, College Station, TX 77843-4474, USA
E-mail address: jrdavidson@cvm.tamu.edu

Vet Clin Small Anim 45 (2015) 537–564
http://dx.doi.org/10.1016/j.cvsm.2015.01.009
0195-5616/15/$ – see front matter © 2015 Elsevier Inc. All rights reserved.

Box 1
Initial wound management

- Cover wound with clean bandage
- Address potentially life-threatening conditions (eg, shock)
- Sedate or anesthetize when patient is stable
- Cover wound surface with sterile, water-soluble gel
- Surgically clip hair with wide margin around wound for bandage to adhere well
- Irrigate the wound with balanced electrolyte solution, avoiding high pressure
- Consider surgical debridement, but avoid if there is any question
- Bandage with a semiocclusive dressing

---

sedation or general anesthesia, which may need to be delayed until patients have been stabilized. Definitive wound management should begin as soon as patients are stable. The skin adjacent to an open wound should be prepared as for aseptic surgery. However, the surgical scrub detergents are cytotoxic and should not be allowed to contact the wound surface. Whenever the wound is uncovered, the principles of strict aseptic technique should be followed. At a minimum, involved personnel should wear surgical masks and sterile gloves to avoid further contaminating the wound, particularly in the early stages of healing.

DEBRIDEMENT

The focus of initial wound care is to reduce the presence of foreign material, bacterial load, and damaged or necrotic tissue. The presence of these substances can provide a focus for infection, prolong the inflammatory phase of healing, and impede wound contraction and epithelialization. If a wound is minimally contaminated and has healthy tissue, it may be closed after cleaning. If the wound has gross contamination, foreign material, severely damaged tissue, or loss of soft tissues, management as an open wound may be required. The wound may be allowed to heal by second intention or may be closed surgically (as primary closure or by use of grafts or flaps) once the wound bed is composed of healthy, uninfected tissue.

Debridement may be selective or nonselective. Selective debridement generally involves the use of endogenous or exogenous enzymes to remove only debris or damaged tissue while leaving healthy tissue intact. In contrast, during nonselective debridement, some healthy tissue is inadvertently removed along with the necrotic tissue and debris. Nonselective debridement involves physical removal of tissue and debris and is also referred to as mechanical debridement (**Table 1**).

NONSELECTIVE DEBRIDEMENT
Wound Irrigation

Mechanical debridement may be used to clean the wound bed, with the most common method being wound irrigation. The purpose of wound irrigation is to mechanically flush away surface bacteria, foreign material, and necrotic debris. Although it is a nonselective type of debridement, it will not damage healthy tissues if appropriate irrigation solutions and pressures are used. There is no strong evidence that cleansing wounds increases healing or reduces infection, but it is almost universally recommended.[1,2]

Table 1
Methods of nonselective (mechanical) wound debridement

Method of Debridement	Advantages	Disadvantages	Indications
Irrigation	There is rapid removal of surface exudate and contaminants. Tissue damage is minimal if done properly.	Hypotonic or cytotoxic solutions can damage tissue. High-pressure irrigation can damage tissue or force contaminants into deeper tissue layers. It will not remove embedded contaminants or attached necrotic tissue.	It is used to remove wound contaminants. Lavage with copious amounts of fluid is most appropriate in the first few days of wound management.
Surgical excision	It can quickly remove large amounts of necrotic tissue and debris.	Accurate assessment of tissue viability is not always possible. Some viable tissue will likely be removed. Excision may be limited by adjacent structures, (eg, nerves, arteries and tendons) that must be preserved for function.	It is used to remove large areas of obviously necrotic tissue. It is used to remove contaminants that are large enough to be grasped with thumb forceps.
Adherent bandage (eg, wet-to-dry or dry-to-dry)	—	It will remove and/or damage viable tissue. It is uncomfortable for patients to wear. Bandage removal is painful.	It is not recommended.

Balanced electrolyte solutions are preferred for use in wound irrigation (**Table 2**). Tap water is acceptable for the initial wound irrigation, although the hypotonic nature of tap water can cause cell destruction.[3] Antibiotics or antiseptics may be added to the lavage solution. If antiseptics are used, the solution must be created with sufficient dilution in order to minimize tissue injury.[4] No one type of fluid has been shown to be superior in preventing wound infection, and there is some question as to the importance of wound irrigation as a means to reduce infection.[2,5]

A 0.05% chlorhexidine diacetate solution is created using one part of a 2% stock solution to 40 parts of an isotonic fluid, which is equivalent to approximately 25 mL of stock antiseptic solution into 1 L of a balanced electrolyte solution. Chlorhexidine forms precipitate in electrolyte solutions, but this does not reduce its effectiveness.[6] More potent solutions may be cytotoxic and delay granulation tissue formation. Chlorhexidine solution has a broad spectrum of activity, with residual activity, and is not inactivated by organic matter.[7,8]

An alternative solution is 0.1% povidone-iodine solution, which is created by combining 1 part 10% stock solution with 100 parts of an isotonic fluid. This amount

Table 2
Irrigation solutions

Type of Fluid	Examples	Indications
Isotonic fluids	Balanced electrolyte solutions: Lactated Ringer solution Normosol-R (Hospira, Inc, Lake Forest, IL) Plasma-Lyte (Baxter Healthcare Corporation, Deerfield, IL) Unbalanced electrolyte solution: Normal (0.9%) saline	A balanced electrolyte fluid is preferred.
Hypotonic fluids	Tap water Distilled water	Tap water is acceptable for wound irrigation, although it has some cytotoxic effects; prolonged use may delay wound healing. Distilled water is not recommended.
Antiseptic irrigation solutions	0.05% Chlorhexidine diacetate (~25 mL of stock solution per liter of balanced electrolyte solution) 0.1% Povidone-iodine (~10 mL of stock solution per 100 mL of balanced electrolyte solution) 0.01% Chlorhexidine gluconate with tris-EDTA solution	Chlorhexidine diacetate and povidone-iodine solutions must be properly diluted to avoid cytotoxicity. These fluids primarily work by their mechanical action and have no significant advantage over isotonic fluids. Tris-EDTA solution will greatly increase the antimicrobial effectiveness of the solution.
Other irrigation solutions	Hydrogen peroxide Dakin solution Acetic acid	All are cytotoxic. None are recommended.

Abbreviation: EDTA, ethylenediaminetetraacetic acid.

is equivalent to approximately 10 mL of stock antiseptic solution into 1000 mL of a balanced electrolyte solution. Povidone iodine has a wide spectrum of antimicrobial activity; but is inactivated by organic matter, such as blood or exudate. There is also a risk of contact sensitization with povidone iodine. The residual activity of povidone iodine is poor compared with chlorhexidine.[9]

Tris–ethylenediaminetetraacetic acid (EDTA) may be added to lavage solutions to help lyse gram-negative bacteria, such as *Pseudomonas aeruginosa*, *Escherichia coli*, and *Proteus vulgaris*, and may have synergistic effects with certain systemic antibiotics.[7] Tris-EDTA solution may be prepared by adding 1.2 g of EDTA and 6.05 g of tris to 1 L of sterile water. Then sodium is added until the pH is 8, and the solution is autoclaved for 15 minutes. This solution can be added to 0.01% chlorhexidine gluconate solution. Hydrogen peroxide, Dakin solution, and acetic acid all have poor antimicrobial activity, are cytotoxic, and are not recommended for use in open wounds.[10]

The ideal amount of pressure used to flush wounds has not been established. Very high pressures (70 psi), such as that produced by pulsatile lavage instruments, may drive contaminants and debris into loose tissue planes and damage the tissue, which could reduce tissue health and resistance to infection.[8] A common technique is to use a 35-mL syringe with an 18-gauge needle to generate 7 to 8 psi. Low-pressure irrigation can be done by flowing sterile fluid from a drip set spiked into a bag of sterile fluid or pouring fluid from a sterile bottle or by use of a bulb syringe. The level of pressure most appropriate for irrigation is unclear, and no one irrigation technique has been shown to be superior.[11,12] Use of sponges to scrub wounds is not recommended because it will damage tissues, resulting in reduced ability to resist infection.

Surgical Debridement

Surgical debridement is indicated for removing large amounts of necrotic debris. Sterile instruments, electrosurgery, or surgical laser may be used for surgical debridement. Aseptic technique must be used to prevent iatrogenic contamination. Foreign debris that was not removed by wound irrigation may be removed with thumb forceps. Excessive removal of healthy tissue should be avoided because it may delay wound healing and make closure more difficult.

Tissue viability can be difficult to determine during the preliminary wound assessment, so initial tissue debridement should be conservative. Tissue that is obviously necrotic should be excised, but tissue with questionable viability should be reassessed at a later day (**Box 2**). Necrotic skin may be black, although normal pigmentation can obfuscate this assessment. Severe skin contusions may recover or may progress to necrosis. Lack of bleeding when the skin edge is cut may indicate congestion and does not consistently predict skin viability. Conversely, bleeding at the skin edge is no guarantee that the tissue will maintain viability over the first few days.

Debridement is begun in the superficial tissues and proceeds to the deeper tissue layers in a stepwise fashion. After excising any necrotic skin, the subcutaneous tissues are assessed for viability and managed accordingly. Subcutaneous tissue that is compromised and contaminated may be excised from the underlying skeletal muscle, taking care to avoid excising fat from the overlying skin. The extent of tissue necrosis is usually apparent within 24 to 48 hours after tissue injury, so repeated debridement may be done as the extent of tissue necrosis becomes more apparent. When managing an open wound, surgical debridement is often done in conjunction with some type of selective debridement (eg, bandages to promote autolytic debridement) to completely rid the wound of contaminants and devitalized tissue.

Gauze Sponges

Mechanical debridement may be accomplished by the use of dry-to-dry or wet-to-dry bandages. A dry-to-dry bandage is applied by placing dry gauze sponges on the wound surface. The sponges absorb serous discharge from the wound and then dry, so tissue and debris on the surface of the wound are physically removed when the bandage is pulled away from the wound. A wet-to-dry bandage is similar, except the gauze sponges contacting the wound surface are moistened to help reduce the viscosity of wound fluid to promote absorption of exudate into the bandage. The gauze dries by the time of bandage removal, which results in adherence to the wound surface and nonselective debridement of tissue and debris as the gauze is removed.

Box 2
Reassess wound

- Sedate or anesthetize patients.

- Involved personnel should wear surgical masks to avoid wound contamination.

- Remove the bandage and clip more hair if needed to keep the wound clean and promote bandage adherence.

- Irrigate to remove any exudate, if it is present.

- Reassess the tissue viability, and surgically debride if necessary.

An unfortunate consequence is removal of some healthy tissue and destruction of epithelial cells. The adherent nature of wet-to-dry and dry-to-dry bandages makes them painful to remove. The open weave of the gauze sponges allows fibers to become embedded in the wound, causing patient discomfort.[13] These gauze bandages also promote dehydration of the wound surface, which results in delayed wound healing.[13,14] In addition, these bandages generally need to be changed 1 to 3 times daily.

Although wet-to-dry and dry-to-dry bandaging were commonly used for wound care in the past, bandaging techniques that use selective debridement are now recommended. Advances in bandage products enable the bandage dressing to maintain a moist wound environment, which results in selective autolytic debridement.[14] These advanced dressings also allow effective gas exchange, enabling improved wound metabolism. In addition, newer bandage materials are more comfortable for patients and require less frequent bandage changes. Healing of chronic wounds has been demonstrated to be superior when advanced dressings are used.[15] Thus, the use of wet-to-dry and dry-to-dry bandages is no longer recommended.

SELECTIVE DEBRIDEMENT
Enzymatic Debridement

Enzymatic debriding agents can be applied to the wound surface to selectively destroy necrotic tissue and liquefy coagulum and bacterial biofilm (**Table 3**). This enzymatic effect allows antibiotics and components of the immune system better access to tissues that are compromised or infected. Enzymatic debridement may be used instead of surgical debridement when patients have a poor anesthetic risk or other surgical contraindication and may also be used as an adjunct to surgical debridement when excision could potentially compromise healthy tissues that must be preserved for adequate reconstruction or functional outcome.

Enzymatic agents are available as ointments or gels containing streptokinase, trypsin, fibrinolysin, protease, or collagenase.[16] Enzymatic debridement can be slow and expensive. Its use may be limited in the treatment of large areas. Ideally, enzymatic debridement is selective and occurs without pain or bleeding. However, it can damage or dehydrate normal tissue. Enzymatic debridement can cause collagenase and fibrinolysin to inhibit the cellular products needed for wound repair, thus delaying wound healing.[16] In addition, enzymes should be contained within the wound bed because persistent contact with adjacent healthy tissues will result in maceration. The enzyme preparation should be covered by a nonadherent dressing, which should typically be changed in 12 to 24 hours.

Biosurgical Debridement

Medical maggots may be used to debride wounds that are necrotic or infected and are particularly useful when effective surgical debridement is not possible.[17,18] Sterile maggots are bred specifically for this purpose using greenbottle fly (*Phaenicia sericata* or *Lucilia sericata*) larvae. The maggots secrete proteolytic digestive enzymes into the wound and consume up to 75 mg of necrotic tissue per day.[7] This species of maggots will not damage healthy dermis or subcutaneous tissue, although they can destroy healthy epithelium. Maggots have the potential to lyse bacteria, including methicillin-resistant *Staphylococcus aureus*. Biosurgical debridement does not cause bleeding and is associated with minimal or no pain.

Maggots require a certain temperature, oxygen supply, and a moist wound surface, which can be achieved with a cage dressing. A wound dressing, such as a

Table 3
Methods of selective wound debridement

Method of Debridement	Advantages	Disadvantages	Indications
Enzymatic agents (ointments or gels) Accuzyme (Healthpoint Ltd, Blackpoint, England) Granulex (Pfizer, New York City, NY) Collagenase Santyl (Smith & Nephew, London, England)	Minimal tissue damage if done properly Not painful Selective debridement	Slow process May be expensive Can damage normal tissue with prolonged contact Not practical for large wounds	Use instead of surgical debridement, when risk of anesthesia is high Use in regions where surgical excision has risk of compromising healthy structures that are needed for wound reconstruction or functional outcome
Biosurgical Medical maggots (Monarch Labs, Irvine, CA)	Can destroy bacteria Usually nonpainful Selective debridement	Must buy or create cage dressing to contain maggots Can be uncomfortable in some wounds	Same indications as for enzymatic agents
Autolytic debridement (maintain moist wound environment with bandage)	Destroys bacteria Does not damage healthy tissue Bandage not painful or pruritic No pain with bandage removal Infrequent bandage changes Selective debridement	Variety of products available confusing	Any open wound Can be used after wound irrigation or surgical debridement

hydrocolloid, is used to absorb wound secretions at the perimeters of the wound. Maggots are applied directly on the wound at a density of 5 to 8 per square centimeter.[19] The maggots are contained within the wound by lightly covering them with gauze and Dacron chiffon mesh or nylon stocking. Maggots are generally removed within 48 to 72 hours and replaced if needed.

Autolytic Debridement

Autolytic debridement is optimal because healthy tissue is spared. Autolytic debridement occurs when a moist environment is maintained at the wound surface. This moisture allows normal cellular processes to destroy bacteria and remove or repair damaged tissue. Autolytic debridement is promoted by using hydrophilic, occlusive, or semiocclusive bandages, which allow some wound exudate to remain in contact with the wound surface and keep it moist. Wound exudate contains endogenous enzymes, growth factors, and cytokines that stimulate angiogenesis, granulation tissue formation, and epithelialization. White blood cells migrate more readily in a moist environment, so phagocytosis of necrotic debris and bacteria is improved. If patients are receiving systemic antibiotics, they will be present in the wound exudate, helping to prevent or control infection.[8] Bandages also keep the wound surface warm, which enhances enzymatic activity. Moist wounds are less painful and less pruritic than wounds that are allowed to become dry.

Oxygen delivery is important for aerobic metabolism and is needed for formation of granulation tissue, fibroblast formation, wound contraction, and epithelialization. Thus, semiocclusive bandages are generally desirable because they allow gaseous exchange of water and air.

Proper wound preparation is needed to create an optimal environment for autolytic debridement. Autolytic debridement may be inhibited by the presence of large amounts of necrotic tissue. Surgical debridement may be indicated before bandaging if gross contamination or large areas of necrotic tissue are identified. Wound irrigation may be indicated to remove excessive wound exudation and surface contaminants.

An appropriate bandage is required to maintain a moist wound environment that enables autolytic debridement. A moist wound surface is desirable, but the presence of excessive amounts of exudate can separate tissue layers to delay healing.[8] Therefore, wound dressings should absorb excessive exudates, without dehydrating the wound surface. Bandaging the wound also helps maintain normal tissue temperatures, which improves wound blood flow and cellular functions.

The principle of moist wound healing is put into practice by the use of hydrophilic dressings (**Box 3**). The rate of wound exudation often dictates selection of the most

---

Box 3
Types of hydrophilic dressings: promote moist wound environment and autolytic debridement

- Calcium alginate
- Polyurethane foam
- Hydrogel
- Hydrocolloid
- Hydrofiber
- Some topical products (eg, maltodextrin, collagen)

appropriate primary layer of the wound bandage. A wound with minimal exudate may benefit from some form of a hydrogel dressing, which can provide moisture to the wound and maintain a thin film of fluid on the wound surface. For a mild to moderately exudative wound, a hydrocolloid or foam may be more appropriate. These dressings are dry on contact but absorb wound exudate to form a gelatinous layer at the wound surface. Heavily exudative wounds may be dressed with alginate, which absorb copious secretions. Some of these dressings are also available with antimicrobial agents impregnated. Dressings should be maintained by a semiocclusive covering to allow exchange of gases. The bandage dressing should be sterile and applied using aseptic technique. This practice is particularly important before the formation of granulation tissue, when the wound is most susceptible to infection.

ANTIMICROBIALS

Bacterial infection can delay wound healing, so clinically relevant infections should be avoided or eliminated. Most traumatic wounds heal normally without prophylactic antimicrobial treatment. Wounds may be contaminated with microorganisms that are cultured from swabs of the wound surface or exudate, but this is not necessarily a clinical problem.[20] There is debate regarding the use of antibiotics and antiseptics in the treatment of nonhealing wounds that have no clinical signs of infection.[21] Diagnosis of wound infection should be based on culture and sensitivity of samples taken from the deep wound tissue, and these results should inform selection of systemic antibiotics.[20]

There is no consensus regarding when and how infected wounds should be treated. Systemic antimicrobial therapy is indicated for advancing cutaneous infections or infections involving the deeper tissues.[21] Treatment with an antimicrobial that has a narrow spectrum of activity is preferred because prolonged administration of broad-spectrum antibiotics will favor the proliferation of more resistant organisms. Systemic antimicrobial therapy can usually be discontinued once healthy granulation tissue is present, partly because penetration into chronic granulation tissue is limited.[22] Wounds that only have localized signs of infection may be treated by topical methods alone. These methods may include antimicrobial products and antimicrobial bandage dressings, along with bandaging methods to promote moist wound healing. The use of modalities such as hyperbaric oxygen therapy, electrical stimulation, or laser therapy may also be considered.

TOPICAL PRODUCTS

Many topical products are advocated to enhance wound healing (**Table 4**). Most wounds will heal well using basic wound care techniques with proper bandage application. However, various topical products may be considered for patients with chronic, nonhealing wounds or when factors are present that may delay wound healing (**Box 4**). After applying a topical product, a bandage is applied to cover the wound and maintain the product on the wound surface. There is not sufficient evidence in the veterinary literature to make recommendations for or against various topical wound products.[10]

Topical Antimicrobials

Topical treatment with antiseptics, silver-based dressings, hyperosmotic dressings, and other dressings that support autolytic debridement provide broad-spectrum reduction in microbial burden. Additional topical agents may be used early in wound management to reduce contaminating microbes and are preferred over systemic

Table 4
Topical products

Agent	Products Available	Comments
Antibiotics	Triple antibiotic ointment Neosporin (Johnson & Johnson, New Brunswick, NJ) Silver sulfadiazine cream Thermazene cream (Covidien, Minneapolis, MN) Nitrofurazone cream/ointment Gentamycin ointment	Most products have a broad spectrum and may be used in combination with systemic antibiotics. Ointments may prevent tissue desiccation. Some products may delay wound contraction and/or epithelialization.
Tripeptide-copper complex	Iamin hydrating gel (ProCyte, Redmond, WA)	It stimulates granulation tissue in chronic wounds.
Maltodextrin	Maltodextrin gel or powder Multidex (DeRoyal, Powell, TN)	It creates a layer on the wound surface that promotes a moist wound environment. It has antibacterial properties. It promotes autolytic debridement.
Acemannan	Acemannan gel or freeze-dried powder CarraVet gel (CarraVet, Palmetto, GA)	It stimulates early wound healing. It can promote excessive granulation tissue, which inhibits wound contraction.
Aloe vera	Included in commercial lotions and ointments	Antithromboxane and antiprostaglandin properties benefit superficial inflammation (eg, burns). It may not benefit an open wound.
Growth factors	Available in gels or dressings Regranex (Smith & Nephew, London, England)	It stimulates granulation tissue. The use of a single growth factor has questionable value but may benefit a chronic nonhealing wound.
Platelet-rich plasma	Plasma concentrates	It may stimulate chronic wound healing. There is limited evidence, so its use is controversial.

Chitosan	Impregnated in bandage dressing: HemCon bandages (HemCon Medical Technologies, Inc, Portland, OR) Opticell (Medline Industries, Inc, Mundelein, IL)	It enhances the function of inflammatory cells, fibroblasts, and cytokines to stimulate granulation tissue. It is hemostatic.
Collagen	Bovine collagen gel, powder, sheet or sponge Woun'Dres Collagen Hydrogel (Coloplast, Minneapolis, MN) Medifil Collagen particles (Human Biosciences, Inc, Gaithersburg, MD) Puracol Collagen (Medline Industries, Inc) Collasate (PRN Pharmacal, Pensacola, FL) Biostep Collagen Matrix (Smith & Nephew) Fibracol Plus (Systagenix, San Antonio, TX)	It absorbs fluid from highly exudative wounds and maintains a moist wound surface. It promotes autolytic debridement. It provides scaffold for extracellular matrix.
Honey	Raw honey or impregnated in bandage dressing Medihoney (Derma Sciences, Princeton, NJ) TheraHoney sheet (Medline Industries, Inc) TheraHoney foam (Medline Industries, Inc) TheraHoney gel (Medline Industries, Inc)	The hyperosmotic effect dehydrates microorganisms and reduces tissue edema. It is antimicrobial. It stimulates granulation tissue. It is appropriate until granulation tissue is present. The bandage may need frequent changing with a highly exudative wound. Honey bandages may be painful.
Sugar	Granulated sugar	The hyperosmotic effect dehydrates microorganisms. It stimulates tissue granulation tissue but is less effective than honey. The bandage may need to be changed up to 3 times daily. Sugar bandages may be painful.

Box 4
Factors that contribute to delayed wound healing

- Host factors
  - Malnourishment
  - Geriatric
  - Hepatic disease
  - Hyperadrenocorticism
  - Diabetes mellitus
  - Uremia
  - Obesity
- Wound factors
  - Foreign material
  - Infection
  - Antiseptics
  - Lack of warmth
  - Excessive exudate
  - Tissue desiccation
  - Impaired blood supply
- Extrinsic factors
  - Radiation therapy
  - Some chemotherapy
  - Corticosteroids

---

antibiotics. Potential benefits of topical drugs should outweigh their potential cytotoxic effects. A variety of topical antimicrobial agents are available.

A triple antibiotic ointment, containing bacitracin zinc, neomycin sulfate, and polymyxin B sulfate, may be used for a broad-spectrum antimicrobial effect to prevent infection of mildly contaminated wounds. It is not cytotoxic and may enhance wound epithelialization by promoting a moist wound surface, although it may delay wound contraction.[7]

Silver sulfadiazine ointment has been used on burn wounds because of its antibacterial and antifungal effects. However, in a study of partial-thickness burn wounds in people, honey dressings seemed to be superior to silver sulfadiazine ointment.[23] Silver-impregnated dressings may be a better choice than silver sulfadiazine ointment because the dressings are associated with less pain and less frequent bandage changes.[24]

Nitrofurazone has broad-spectrum activity but little effect against *Pseudomonas spp.* Nitrofurazone delays epithelialization,[25] and it has reduced the antibacterial effect in the presence of organic matter.

Gentamicin sulfate is effective against gram-negative bacteria and *Staphylococcus* spp. It is applied as an oil-in-water cream that may inhibit wound contraction and epithelialization.[25,26] However, gentamicin in an isotonic solution does not inhibit contraction and promotes epithelialization.

Tripeptide-Copper Complex

Tripeptide-copper complex has been reported to stimulate neovascularization, collagen deposition, wound contraction, and epithelialization. It may be used in the late inflammatory and early repair phase to stimulate granulation tissue and may be appropriate to stimulate healing of chronic, ischemic open wounds.[27]

Maltodextrin

Maltodextrin is a D-glucose polysaccharide derived from hydrolysis of corn or potato starch. Hydrolysis of maltodextrin may provide a source of glucose to the cells.[8] Maltodextrin may be used to promote healing of slow-healing, infected wounds. It is available in powder or gel form, and it absorbs moisture to form a protective layer on the wound surface to promote a moist wound environment. Maltodextrin reportedly attracts white blood cells and cytokines into the wound and may enhance early granulation tissue formation and epithelialization.[7] It also has antibacterial properties.[7] Maltodextrin must be flushed from the wound surface before reapplication during daily bandage changes.

Acemannan

Acemannan is derived from the aloe vera plant.[28] It is available as a topical wound hydrogel or freeze-dried gel form. Acemannan has hydrophilic properties that promote a moist wound environment. It enhances the early stages of wound healing by serving as a growth factor and increasing cytokine levels. Acemannan stimulates macrophages, angiogenesis, and epidermal growth but can also cause excess granulation tissue, which inhibits wound contraction.[7,8]

Growth Factors

Growth factors are naturally occurring hormones that cause cellular growth and regulate the wound healing process. Platelet-derived growth factor is available as a gel, and epidermal growth factor has been incorporated in a wound dressing.[29] Because the healing process is dynamic and complex, involving multiple endogenous factors at various times, application of a single growth factor is of questionable value.[8]

Platelet-Derived Products

Platelets are a good source of complex growth factors. Commercial products are available that allow veterinarians to harvest and concentrate platelets to produce platelet-rich plasma (PRP). The use of PRP has been shown to enhance fibroblast proliferation and migration and accelerate epithelial differentiation. Gel created from PRP enhanced wound epithelialization in an equine model.[30] It also resulted in faster healing of chronic decubital ulcers in dogs as compared with paraffin-impregnated gauze.[31] Application of autologous PRP gel did not improve wound healing in another equine study.[32] There is currently a lack of evidence to support the use of PRP in chronic wounds in humans.[33] The use of PRP in clinical or contaminated wounds has not been fully evaluated, and its use remains controversial.

Chitosan

Chitosan is a natural biopolymer that is derived from chitin in the exoskeleton of shellfish. It is thought to promote various aspects of wound healing by upregulation of growth factors.[34] Chitosan is biodegradable, biocompatible, nontoxic, nonantigenic, and antimicrobial.[35] It may also be used to help achieve hemostasis following surgical debridement. Fatal hemorrhagic pneumonia has been reported in dogs that were administered more than 50 mg/kg subcutaneously. Various wound products contain chitosan embedded in the dressing.[36]

Collagen

Collagen products are available in sheet, powder, or sponge form. Collagen is hydrophilic, which helps maintain a moist wound environment for autolytic debridement[37]; it may also provide substrate for fibroblasts. Collagen also has hemostatic properties, so may be used after surgical debridement. Collagen can serve as a scaffold to facilitate wound healing, with the collagen fibrils providing a network for fibroblast migration.[7] Collagen has been used to promote granulation and epithelialization, particularly in chronic wounds with delayed healing.

Honey

Honey is available as raw honey in tubes or jars or impregnated in dressings. Honey enhances wound debridement, reduces edema and inflammation, and promotes granulation tissue formation and epithelialization.[7] It accelerates collagen maturation and maintains optimal pH conditions for fibroblast activity. Honey is purported to contain amino acids, vitamins, sugars, and trace elements that stimulate tissue growth.[8] Honey has an osmotic effect that dehydrates microorganisms, but the antimicrobial effects of honey cannot be explained by hyperosmolality alone. Low pH, phytochemicals, and the release of small amounts of hydrogen peroxide and methylglyoxal also contribute to its antimicrobial properties.[38,39] Because honey is a natural product, its effectiveness may vary with the source of the product and the processing methods used. Therefore, use of medicinal honey is recommended; medical-grade honey is rated according to its antimicrobial properties. Manuka honey, derived from the flowers of the tea tree, is considered to be the most effective honey.[7]

Honey dressings may be used in the inflammatory and early repair phases of healing and is discontinued when debridement is complete and healthy granulation tissue is present.[8] Gauze soaked in honey may be used as a primary bandage layer. The osmotic action of the honey draws fluid from the tissues, which may be painful. A honey-soaked gauze dressing may need to be replaced 1 to 3 times daily for highly exudative wounds because the exudate will dilute the honey and diminish its osmotic effects. If the wound produces a small amount of exudate, the honey dressing may be changed in 1 to 3 days. Honey is water soluble, so it is flushed from the wound during dressing changes.

When using a honey-soaked gauze, the gauze may adhere to viable tissues, causing pain and irritation during removal. This effect may be avoided by adhering to the principles of moist wound healing and using commercial hydrophilic dressings that are impregnated with honey.

Sugar

Sugar has hypertonic effects similar to honey, which dehydrates microorganisms and inhibits their growth.[7] Sugar is primarily used during the inflammatory stage of wound healing. Sugar may also enhance granulation tissue formation and epithelialization but does not have the same inherent antiinflammatory and wound stimulation effects as honey.[8] Sugar is applied in a 1-cm thick layer on the wound surface and covered by an absorbent bandage.[7] Bandage changes are typically required 2 to 3 times daily to maintain the osmolality of the wound. Application of sugar is reportedly uncomfortable for some human patients. There are very few studies on the use of sugar in wound management; it has been advocated for use in human medicine in remote areas or disaster situations, when medical resources are limited.[40,41]

BANDAGING TO PROMOTE MOIST WOUND HEALING

Bandages are used to support the tissues, protect the wound from external trauma and contamination, and promote wound healing. In addition, the bandage can apply pressure to control hemorrhage or help obliterate dead space. The outer layers of the bandage function to absorb wound exudate, stabilize the tissue, and maintain the dressing in position over the wound. The portion of the bandage that contacts the wound is called the primary layer but may also be referred to as the dressing.

There are several advanced wound dressings, which interact with the wound surface to enhance healing.[13,20] The dressing may perform several functions, including absorption of wound exudate, transfer of exudate to the secondary layer, maintain a moist wound environment, facilitate wound debridement, deliver a product to promote healing, and reduce bacterial numbers. The most appropriate material for the primary layer varies with the stage of wound healing (**Table 5**) and the amount of exudate. No single dressing is suitable for all types of wounds, and there is no perfect dressing (**Box 5**). A hydrophilic dressing is one that attracts fluid and maintains a moist environment at the wound surface (see **Box 3**). Hydrophilic dressings should be made to fit completely within the wound bed to avoid maceration of adjacent skin.

Time between bandage changes depends on the type of dressing and the amount of wound exudate. For a noninfected wound, hydrophilic dressings generally need to

Table 5
Stages of wound healing

Stage or Phase	Approximate Time	Characteristics	Goal of Bandage
Inflammatory	0–5 d	Inflammatory cells eliminate contaminants and nonviable tissue. Platelets release growth factors to attract fibroblasts, which produce fibrin and collagen. Fluid extravasation may cause edema.	Maintain a moist wound environment to promote autolytic debridement. Protect the wound from external contaminants. Provide support to tissues.
Repair	5–21 d	Inflammatory cells and mediators diminish. Collagen and neovascularization form granulation tissue, which provides a barrier to infection. Epithelialization may begin once there is granulation tissue. Myofibroblasts in granulation tissue cause wound contraction.	Maintain a moist wound environment to stimulate granulation tissue, epithelialization, and wound contraction. Bandage may need to support tissues, depending on location and severity of tissue damage.
Maturation	21 d to weeks or months	Collagen reorganizes and forms cross-links to strengthen the tissue. Tissue structures are reformed.	Wound is typically no longer open and has contracted/epithelialized. Bandage is no longer needed, unless to support weakened tissues.

Box 5
Characteristics of an optimal wound dressing

- Maintains moist wound environment that supports selective autolytic debridement, granulation, epithelialization, and/or contraction
- Low adherence to wound surface
- Provides mechanical protection
- Requires infrequent changes
- Cost-efficient
- Provides thermal insulation
- Absorbs excess exudate and blood at wound surface
- Protects wound from external contaminants
- Adequate gaseous exchange
- Nontoxic, nonirritating
- Easy to change
- Conforms well to the wound surface

---

be changed every 2 to 3 days during the inflammatory stage and every 4 to 7 days during the repair phase. Dressing changes are needed more frequently in infected wounds than noninfected wounds. Each time the bandage is changed, the wound should be assessed to determine the most appropriate wound dressing (**Table 6**). If the dressing seems to have additional capacity to absorb exudate, the outer layers of the bandage may be changed without disturbing the dressing.

Nonadherent Dressings

Nonadherent dressings are most commonly used over a healthy wound or skin graft to enable bandage removal with minimal disruption of the underlying tissue. They may be composed of mesh fabric impregnated with paraffin or petrolatum. Another type of nonadherent dressing is composed of a thin layer of absorbent cotton fibers enclosed in a perforated plastic film. Both allow transfer of tissue fluids through the dressing to an overlying absorptive layer of the bandage and can speed the rate of wound epithelialization.[42–44]

Hypertonic Saline

Hypertonic dressings (20% saline-soaked sponges) use the osmotic gradient to lyse and destroy bacterial cells.[7] However, this may also destroy fibroblasts, thus slowing wound healing. The hyperosmotic effect removes exudate and accompanying debris from the wound and reduces surrounding tissue edema.[7] This same osmotic effect can dehydrate viable tissue if the dressing is left in place too long. Hypertonic saline dressings are indicated for necrotic, infected wounds with heavy exudates. The osmotic action desiccates bacteria and necrotic tissue.

Hydrogel

Hydrogel preparations are available as water- or glycerin-based amorphous gels, impregnated gauze, or sheet dressings. Hydrogels are hydrophilic, insoluble dressings made primarily from synthetic polymers. Hydrogels help maintain a moist wound environment that promotes debridement, granulation tissue, and epithelialization.[42]

Because of their high water content, they do not absorb large amounts of exudate; so they should be reserved for less exudative wounds. Hydrogels can also be used to rehydrate dry wound beds. They are nonadherent and provide some pain relief. Sheet dressings should be cut to the size of the open wound to prevent maceration of the skin at the wound edges. Hydrogel may be used to promote autolytic debridement during the inflammatory stage of wound healing and can also be used over granulation tissue to promote epithelialization and contraction.[8,14]

Foam Dressings

Foam dressings are composed of absorbent, nonirritating synthetic polymer, such as polyurethane foam. They create a moist environment to promote granulation and epithelialization.[14] Foam dressings provide thermal insulation to the wound. Foam dressings are nonadherent to the wound surface, but some products have adhesive borders that adhere to normal adjacent skin. Foam products vary in conformability and absorbency. However, foam products absorb light to heavy amounts of exudate; so they are most suited for highly exudative wounds. In wounds with minimal exudate, foam may be moistened before application. The dressing should be changed when absorbed fluid comes within 1 in of the foam edge.[45]

Hydrocolloid

Hydrocolloid dressings are occlusive or semiocclusive dressings composed of biocompatible hydrophilic polymers, such as carboxymethylcellulose with gelatins or pectin.[20] Hydrocolloid products are available as powders, pastes, or sheets. As the hydrocolloid absorbs wound exudate, it liquefies to form a viscous gel on the wound surface.[37] This gel provides a moist wound environment that enables autolytic debridement. The surrounding skin should be protected from hydrocolloid pads to prevent maceration. Hydrocolloids may contain an occlusive outer covering that prevents water vapor exchange between the wound and air; however, as the gel forms it becomes progressively more permeable. Hydrocolloids are primarily used for superficial wounds with minimal exudate to promote granulation or epithelialization.[20] Absorbency is low to moderate, depending on the composition of the product. Hydrocolloid pads contour easily, but their relative stiffness may impede wound contraction. Some hydrocolloid dressings have a self-adhering border and can be applied without a secondary dressing. However, adherence can be a problem in dogs and cats; so a light bandage may be needed to hold the hydrocolloid in place. Hydrocolloid sheets should be changed when the sheet feels like a fluid-filled blister. When changing the dressing, any gel is flushed from the wound surface before applying a new dressing.

Hydrofiber

Hydrofiber dressings are nonwoven pads or ribbons composed of sodium carboxymethylcellulose fibers.[20] They are essentially hydrocolloid dressings in the form of a hydrophilic nonwoven sheet of fibers. They conform well and are very absorbent. Fluid absorption occurs vertically only, so no fluid should travel horizontally.[20] The advantage of the vertical absorption is that maceration of wound margins is avoided. Hydrofiber products may be used for very exudative wounds and will promote wound cleansing and granulation tissue formation.[20] They should not be used on dry wounds because they are designed to interact with wound exudate to form a gel on the wound surface. Hydrofiber dressings may be left in place for several days, depending on the amount of exudate.

Table 6
Bandage dressings

Dressing	Products Available	Indications
Nonadherent	Fabric impregnated with paraffin or petrolatum Cotton within perforated plastic film Adaptic (Systagenix, San Antonio, TX) Telfa (Covidien, Minneapolis, MN)	Prevent adherence of overlying bandage Allows transfer of exudate into overlying bandage Wound exudate: minimal Stage of healing: repair; also for partial-thickness skin wounds or to cover healing grafts or sutured wounds
Hypertonic saline	Hypertonic saline-impregnated gauze Curasalt (Covidien)	Good for highly contaminated or infected wounds; hyperosmotic effect dehydrates microorganisms and reduces tissue edema Can be used to debride an eschar Caution: can dehydrate wound and adjacent tissues if left in place too long for the amount of exudate Wound exudate: moderate to copious Stage of healing: inflammatory
Hydrogel	Gel, impregnated gauze, sheet Curafil Amorphous Gel (Covidien) Curafil Hydrogel Impregnated Gauze (Covidien) Curagel Hydrogel Dressing (Covidien) Carrasyn Hydrogel (Medline Industries, Inc, Mundelein, IL) CarraDres Clear Hydrogel Sheets (Medline Industries, Inc) Tegagel Hydrogel (3M, St Paul, MN)	Can rehydrate wound or prevent desiccation Caution: may macerate periwound skin Exudate: may be odiferous and yellow and should not be misinterpreted as evidence of infection Wound exudate: minimal or none Stage of healing: inflammatory or repair; good for partial-thickness wounds
Polyurethane foam	Sheet Kendall Foam Wound Dressing (Covidien) Hydrasorb Foam (Covidien) Allevyn Foam (Smith & Nephew, London, England)	Good thermal insulation Wound exudate: moderate to copious; can use on dry wound, if premoistened Caution: can dehydrate wound if left in place too long for the amount of exudate Stage of healing: inflammatory
Hydrocolloid	Powder, paste, or sheet DuoDERM (ConvaTec, Skillman, NJ) Medihoney Hydrocolloid Dressing (Derma Sciences, Princeton, NJ) Nu-Derm Hydrocolloid Wound Dressing (Systagenix, San Antonio, TX) 3M Tegaderm Hydrocolloid Wound Dressing (3M)	Caution: may macerate periwound skin May inhibit wound contraction Exudate: may be odiferous and yellow and should not be misinterpreted as evidence of infection Wound exudate: minimal to moderate Stage of healing: inflammatory or repair

Type	Products	Notes
Hydrofiber	Sheet or rope Aquacel (ConvaTec)	Vertical absorption of fluid to prevent maceration of adjacent tissue Wound exudate: moderate to copious Stage of healing: inflammatory
Alginate	Sheet or rope Curasorb Zinc Calcium Alginate (Covidien) Medihoney Calcium Alginate (Derma Sciences) Maxorb Extra (Medline Industries, Inc) Nu-Derm Alginate (Systagenix) Sorbsan Alginate (Pharma-Plast Ltd, Deeside, UK) 3M Tegaderm Alginate (3M) 3M Tegagen (3M)	Hemostatic, so consider after surgical debridement Caution: can dehydrate wound if left in place too long for the amount of exudate, so avoid over exposed bone or tendon Exudate: may be odiferous and yellow and should not be misinterpreted as evidence of infection Exudate: moderate to copious Stage of healing: inflammatory
Transparent film (semiocclusive)	Adhesive, semipermeable, polyurethane membrane Polyskin II (Covidien) Opsite (Smith & Nephew) 3M Tegaderm Transparent Film (3M)	May have adhesive borders that enable it to be used alone or to cover and maintain the position of a different dressing (eg, hydrogel, foam, hydrocolloid) Caution: waterproof and does not absorb wound fluids, so must be changed if fluid accumulates underneath; may also promote bacterial growth Exudate: minimal or none Stage of healing: partial-thickness skin wounds or sutured wounds
Antimicrobial	PHMB impregnated in dressings, gauze sponges, or roll gauze Kendall AMD Antimicrobial Foam (Covidien) Kerlix AMD Rolls (Covidien) Kerlix AMD Super Sponges (Covidien) Kerlix AMD Gauze Dressing (Covidien) Telfa AMD Dressing (Covidien) May incorporate silver in various forms in various types of bandage dressings (eg, foam, alginate, hydrofiber) Aquacel Ag: hydrofiber dressing (Convatec) Silvasorb wound gel (Medline Industries, Inc) Opticell Ag (Medline Industries, Inc) Biostep Ag Collagen Matrix (Smith & Nephew) Acticoat (Smith & Nephew) Silvercel Nonadherent (Systagenix) Actisorb Silver 220 (Systagenix)	May use PHMB-impregnated roll gauze in outer layers of bandage to maintain dressing in place over wound Both PHMB and silver products: broad-spectrum antimicrobial activity to resist infection Caution: silver dressings may cause green exudate that should not be mistaken for *Pseudomonas* infection Exudate: depends on composition of base dressing Stage of healing: all

Abbreviation: PHMB, polyhexamethylene biguanide.

Alginate Dressings

Alginates are composed of natural polysaccharide fibers or are derived from algae.[20] They are available as soft, nonwoven fibers in the form of sheets or rope. Alginate products conform to the wound and absorb exudate to form a hydrophilic gel-like substance, which contains the bacteria and wound debris and maintains a moist wound environment.[20] Alginates absorb 20 to 30 times their weight, so they are useful for moderately exudative wounds.[20] Depending on the product, the dressing may supply calcium, zinc, or manganese to the wound fluid. Silver ions have also been added to some alginate dressings to enhance antibacterial properties. Alginates have a hemostatic effect, so are suitable for use following surgical debridement. Alginate products are often useful in the early management of wounds, when there is excessive exudate and hemorrhage.[20] An absorbent bandage layer should be applied over the alginate to help retain the wound drainage. Alginate products may be left on the wound for several days, to avoid disturbing the healing tissues. When changing the bandage, the alginate gel is lifted from the wound or flushed with normal saline, which causes minimal wound disruption. Any fragments of alginate left in the wound are broken into calcium and simple sugars, and will not elicit a foreign body reaction. A gel will not form in a dry wound, so alginate should be avoided or should be premoistened for use on minimally exudative wounds. Alginate bandages may remain in place for 1 to 7 days or until drainage is seen on the outer dressing.

Transparent Films

Transparent films are adhesive, semipermeable, polyurethane membrane dressings. They are waterproof and impermeable to contaminants and bacteria but permit transfer of water vapor and atmospheric gases.[7] They have no ability to absorb drainage and need to be changed when fluid accumulates underneath. Their ability to trap moisture could promote the proliferation of skin organisms under the film. Because they are transparent, wounds can be assessed without removing the dressing. Some films have a thin, nonadherent contact layer with an adhesive border. They may be used as a primary layer over partial-thickness wounds or sutured incisions; but use of the film alone should be avoided in the presence of infection, necrotic tissue, or highly exudative wounds.[7] Transparent films are also used as a secondary dressing to protect and secure a primary wound dressing, such as hydrogel sheets, foams, or hydrocolloids. Adhesive films will adhere more readily if the hair is removed and the skin is clean and dry. The film does not adhere well to mobile regions or areas with skin folds.

Antimicrobial Dressings

Polyhexamethylene biguanide (PHMB) is an antibacterial substance that is present in some wound dressings and bandage materials. PHMB has antimicrobial action against gram-positive and gram-negative bacteria and has no apparent negative effects on wound healing.[1] Products containing PHMB resist bacterial colonization on wounds and have prolonged local activity. In addition, gauze rolls impregnated with PHMB may be used in the secondary layer of the bandage to reduce existing microbial burden and protect the wound from further contamination.[46]

Wound products may contain silver in the form of silver ions, elementary silver, nanocrystalline silver, or inorganic silver complexes. Ionic silver-impregnated dressings are available in a variety of formulations, including foam, alginate, polyester mesh, and carboxymethylcellulose fiber dressings. Silver ions may be attached to the wound dressing or may be released into the gel that is produced after contacting the wound exudate. Silver ions form complexes with bacterial proteins, which irreversibly damage the bacteria.[20] Silver dressings have antimicrobial activity against a range of aerobic and anaerobic bacteria, including antibiotic-resistant strains.[47,48] Silver dressings may cause the wound to produce a green exudate resembling that seen with *Pseudomonas* infections, so the exudate must be flushed from the wound before evaluating the wound bed.

OTHER THERAPIES

In most cases, appropriate debridement with proper bandaging results in adequate wound healing. The wound should be closed when it seems healthy and free of infection, unless adequate wound closure by contraction and epithelialization is anticipated. New modalities are always being developed in attempts to hasten healing. Adjunctive therapies may be most beneficial for chronic wounds or when delayed healing is anticipated (see **Box 4**). Physical modalities, such as extracorporeal shock wave, laser, electrical stimulation, or therapeutic ultrasound typically need to be applied to an uncovered wound. When these treatments are desired, they can be administered at the time of a bandage change.

Hyperbaric Oxygen

Chronic nonhealing wounds are frequently hypoxic because of poor perfusion.[21] Low oxygen tension has also been recorded in infected and traumatized tissue. Oxygen is essential for cell growth, wound healing, and resistance to infection. Increased oxygen delivery to the tissues results in angiogenesis and improved immune function.

Hyperbaric oxygen therapy (HBOT) is the inhalation of pure oxygen at a pressure greater than 1 atm. This therapy greatly increases the amount of dissolved oxygen in plasma, resulting in increased tissue oxygen tension. HBOT seems to improve the healing of diabetes-related foot ulcers in people, but there is insufficient evidence to support or refute its effect on other wounds.[49] There are no prospective randomized controlled studies on the indications for HBOT in veterinary medicine.[50] Extrapolating from human medicine, HBOT may be beneficial for necrotizing soft tissue infections or thermal burns.[50]

HBOT chambers are available in various sizes, with some designed specifically for small animals and others designed for equine patients. Veterinary personnel with training in hyperbaric medicine should monitor patients during each therapy session. Hyperbaric chambers are not readily available to most practitioners and can be cost prohibitive.

Potential contraindications for HBOT include pneumothorax, pulmonary disease, history of thoracic or ear surgery, fever, and pregnancy. Complications of HBOT include barotrauma, cataracts, pulmonary dyspnea, and seizures.[50,51]

Extracorporeal Shock Wave Therapy

Extracorporeal shock wave therapy (ESWT) is the delivery of high-energy waves through the tissues. ESWT has been used to suppress exuberant granulation tissue in an equine model to improve wound healing.[52] It has also been shown to increase the rate of epithelialization in both equine and porcine models.[53,54] There is no consensus on the optimal therapeutic protocol regarding duration, strength, or number of pulses; but treatments in humans are commonly administered once or twice weekly, using low or medium energy. A systematic review of the literature concluded that ESWT is a safe, mostly painless adjunctive therapy for wounds in humans; but further studies are needed to evaluate its efficacy and cost-effectiveness.[55]

Laser Therapy

Laser therapy may aid healing of open wounds (**Box 6**).[56–58] However, higher doses of laser can inhibit wound healing or even create cellular damage. Therapeutic laser is typically performed using a wavelength range of 630 nm (visible light) to 904 nm (infrared), with between 1 and 15 W of power. One of the difficulties in evaluating the literature is that the type of laser and therapeutic protocols may vary greatly between studies. In addition, most studies on wound healing have been done in vitro or in vivo on humans, whose skin characteristics are quite different than furred animals. Some studies indicate beneficial effects, whereas others suggest no benefit.[59,60] Laser therapy may have the most promise for wounds with impaired healing properties.

Therapeutic lasers are readily available, with various brands being marketed to the veterinary community. The general guideline for laser treatment is 2 to 6 J/cm^2 once daily for 7 to 10 days for acute wounds and 2 to 8 J/cm^2 once daily for chronic wounds.[61] However, optimal dosages are not known and may vary depending on the wavelength. The laser head should not contact the wound and should be cleaned before and after treatment. There are some cautions for the use of laser therapy (**Table 7**). Hospital personnel can be trained to use the laser and must also be trained with respect to laser safety. All individuals in the room (including patients) must wear protective eyeglasses.

Electrical Stimulation

Several types of transcutaneous electrical stimulation have been used to promote wound healing.[62,63]

Microcurrent electrical stimulation uses continuous or pulsed electrical current waveforms in the microamperage range (1 to 999 μA) to accelerate healing of chronic wounds that have delayed healing.[64] The value of microcurrent electrical stimulation is based on the theory that normal tissue healing is partially mediated by endogenous bioelectrical signals, so the therapy is designed to enhance that effect. When the anode (+) is placed on a moist sterile gauze over the wound bed, with the cathode (−) on the adjacent skin, negatively charged cells (macrophages and neutrophils) will migrate toward the anode, thus promoting the inflammatory stage of wound healing.[64] If the cathode is placed over the wound bed with the anode on the adjacent skin, positively charged cells (fibroblasts, keratinocytes, epidermal cells) will migrate toward the cathode.[64] Thus electrode placement may need to be planned based on the stage of wound healing, or the polarity may be reversed every 3 to 4 treatments to balance the migration of positively and negatively charged cells. There is limited evidence to suggest that an electrical current may inhibit microbial growth, with either

---

Box 6
Potential effects of laser on wound healing

- Accelerate angiogenesis
- Stimulate fibroblasts
- Promote collagen formation
- Enhance production of adenosine triphosphate, protein, and growth factors
- Cause vasodilation
- Improve lymphatic drainage

Table 7
Potential risks associated with laser therapy

Potential Effect/Risk	Recommendation
Retinal damage	Do not treat near the eyes.
	All individuals present must wear eyewear that is protective for the specific wavelength being used.
	Therapy should be delivered in a closed room without windows to avoid accidental exposure to others.
	Beware that laser light may reflect off smooth surfaces.
Darkly pigmented skin, tattoos, and hair can absorb more laser light	Adjust treatment settings to avoid burning hair or skin. Hair may need to be removed if it prevents the laser light from reaching the targeted tissue.
Stimulate cellular activity	Avoid treating over the infected area.
	Avoid treating directly over a malignant lesion.
Alter cellular activity	Avoid using it directly over testicles.
	Avoid using it over thyroid gland.
Vasodilation	Avoid using it over hemorrhagic tissue.

the anode or the cathode over the wound bed. The wound may be treated for 30 to 60 minutes, 2 or 3 times daily, 5 to 7 days per week. There is some evidence to justify the use of microcurrent therapy to treat chronic dermal ulcers in humans.[64]

High-voltage pulsed current therapy (HVPC) is another type of electrical stimulation advocated as an adjunctive treatment of chronic, nonhealing wounds.[64–67] The rationale for its use is the same as for microcurrent electrical stimulation. The suggestions for electrode placement are the same as for microcurrent therapy. There is no evidence to suggest that one polarity is better than the other or that continuous delivery is better than pulsed mode. The voltage amplitude is set between 150 and 250 V, using a frequency between 0.1 and 200 pulses per second. There are some potential contraindications to the use of HVPC (**Table 8**). The wound may be treated for 30 to 90 minutes, once daily, 5 to 7 days per week. There is some evidence to justify the use of HVPC to treat dermal wounds in humans.[64]

Therapeutic Ultrasound

Therapeutic ultrasound is the delivery of acoustic or mechanical energy waves through the tissues. Ultrasound may have a stimulating effect on cells during the inflammatory stage of wound healing, and may also increase collagen strength.[68–71]

Table 8
Potential risks associated with HVPC therapy

Potential Effect/Risk	Recommendation
Increased blood flow	Avoid using it over malignancies.
	Avoid using it over hemorrhagic tissue.
Electrical current	Avoid using it over pacemakers.
	Use it with caution over the ventral neck (vagus nerve, carotid sinuses).
	Use with caution over thorax, especially if patients have cardiac disease.
	Avoid using it over the head, particularly in patients with seizures.

Table 9
Potential risks associated with conventional therapeutic ultrasound

Potential Effect/Risk	Recommendation
Increased blood flow	Tumor growth may be promoted, so avoid using over malignancies. Hemorrhagic response may be enhanced, so use caution over hemorrhagic areas. Use caution with use over infected region because blood flow may spread the infection.
Interfere with electronics	Avoid using over pacemakers
Retinal damage	Avoid using it over the eyes, especially if using ultrasound thermal effects.

Conventional ultrasound therapy is characterized by ultrasonic energy delivered at high frequency (3 MHz) and intensity (0.1–3.0 W/cm^2).[64] The energy is delivered to the tissue through a hand piece that contacts the skin. Transmission of ultrasound energy is improved by use of a coupling medium (typically ultrasound gel) applied to the skin surface to interface with the handpiece. Ultrasound has both thermal and mechanical effects within the tissues that may promote wound healing. The ultrasound energy can be delivered continuously or in a pulsed mode. The pulsed mode may be preferred if the intent is to cause more mechanical than thermal effects. There are some potential risks associated with therapeutic ultrasound, particularly related to the thermal effects (**Table 9**). A typical treatment would be the application of ultrasound for 5 to 10 minutes every other day. There is some evidence to justify the use of conventional ultrasound in the treatment of dermal ulcers in humans.[64]

The MIST therapy system (Celleration Inc, Eden Prairie, MN) is ultrasonic energy that is delivered at a much lower frequency (40 kHz) than conventional ultrasound.[64] It is indicated for cleaning or debriding wounds that contain fibrin, exudates, or bacteria and may also promote healing of chronic wounds.[72–74] A mist of sterile saline transfers ultrasonic energy to the wound bed without direct contact by the handpiece. The energy is delivered in continuous mode. A typical treatment would be the application of ultrasound for 5 to 10 minutes daily. The MIST therapy system seems to have merit for debriding open wounds and promoting wound healing but may not be cost-effective for veterinary use.

SUMMARY

Most wounds will heal without complications. The goals of open wound management are to protect the wound from additional contamination and to maintain a moist wound environment, which is optimal for infection control and wound healing. Conservative surgical debridement may be indicated to remove large areas of necrotic tissue or gross contamination. Wound irrigation is also performed to remove excessive exudation or unattached foreign materials. These nonselective debridement techniques are used in conjunction with hydrophilic bandage dressings that promote selective wound debridement. Dressing selection is based on the stage of wound healing and the amount of exudate, so the most appropriate dressing will change as the wound heals.

Care of chronic nonhealing wounds is more complex. Advanced wound dressings that create a moist wound environment are still indicated. A topical product may be considered, although most have limited evidence supporting their efficacy. The appropriate use of systemic or topical antibiotics and topic antiseptics also remains controversial. In addition, some physical modalities show promise as adjunctive therapy and warrant further investigation.

REFERENCES

1. Atiyeh BS, Dibo SA, Hayek SN. Wound cleansing, topical antiseptics and wound healing. Int Wound J 2009;6:420–30.
2. Fernandez R, Griffiths R. Water for wound cleansing. Cochrane Database Syst Rev 2012;(2):CD003861.
3. Buffa EA, Lubbe AM, Verstraete FJ, et al. The effects of wound lavage solutions on canine fibroblasts: an in vitro study. Vet Surg 1997;26:460–6.
4. Sanchez IR, Nusbaum KE, Swaim SF, et al. Chlorhexidine diacetate and povidone-iodine cytotoxicity to canine embryonic fibroblasts and Staphylococcus aureus. Vet Surg 1988;17:182–5.
5. Khan MN, Naqvi AH. Antiseptics, iodine, povidone iodine and traumatic wound cleansing. J Tissue Viability 2006;16:6–10.
6. Lozier S, Pope E, Berg J. Effects of four preparations of 0.05% chlorhexidine diacetate on wound healing in dogs. Vet Surg 1992;21:107–12.
7. Pavletic MM. Atlas of small animal wound management and reconstructive surgery. 3rd edition. Ames, IA: Wiley-Blackwell; 2010.
8. Hedlund C. Surgery of the integumentary system. In: Fossum TW, editor. Small animal surgery. 3rd edition. St Louis (MO): Mosby Elsevier; 2007. p. 159–259.
9. Jarral OA, McCormack DJ, Ibrahim S, et al. Should surgeons scrub with chlorhexidine or iodine prior to surgery? Interact Cardiovasc Thorac Surg 2011;12:1017–21.
10. Fahie MA, Shettko D. Evidence-based wound management: a systematic review of therapeutic agents to enhance granulation and epithelialization. Vet Clin North Am Small Anim Pract 2007;37:559–77.
11. Chatterjee JS. A critical review of irrigation techniques in acute wounds. Int Wound J 2005;2:258–65.
12. Owens BD, White DW, Wenke JC. Comparison of irrigation solutions and devices in a contaminated musculoskeletal wound survival model. J Bone Joint Surg Am 2009;91:92–8.
13. Mayet N, Choonara YE, Kumar P, et al. A comprehensive review of advanced biopolymeric wound healing systems. J Pharm Sci 2014;103:2211–30.
14. Boateng JS, Matthews KH, Stevens HN, et al. Wound healing dressings and drug delivery systems: a review. J Pharm Sci 2008;97:2892–923.
15. Heyer K, Augustin M, Protz K, et al. Effectiveness of advanced versus conventional wound dressings on healing of chronic wounds: systematic review and meta-analysis. Dermatology 2013;226:172–84.
16. Alford CG, Caldwell FJ. Equine distal limb wounds: new and emerging treatments. Compend Contin Educ Vet 2012;34:E1–6.
17. Armstrong DG, Mossel J, Short B, et al. Maggot debridement therapy: a primer. J Am Podiatr Med Assoc 2002;92:398–401.
18. Falch BM, de Weerd L, Sundsfjord A. Maggot therapy in wound management. Tidsskr Nor Laegeforen 2009;129:1864–7 [in Norwegian].
19. MonarchLabs. Available at: http://www.monarchlabs.com. Accessed October 30, 2014.
20. Dissemond J, Augustin M, Eming SA, et al. Modern wound care - practical aspects of non-interventional topical treatment of patients with chronic wounds. J Dtsch Dermatol Ges 2014;12:541–54.

21. Bowler PG, Duerden BI, Armstrong DG. Wound microbiology and associated approaches to wound management. Clin Microbiol Rev 2001;14:244–69.
22. Robson MC, Edstrom LE, Krizek TJ, et al. The efficacy of systemic antibiotics in the treatment of granulating wounds. J Surg Res 1974;16:299–306.
23. Gupta SS, Singh O, Bhagel PS, et al. Honey dressing versus silver sulfadiazine dressing for wound healing in burn patients: a retrospective study. J Cutan Aesthet Surg 2011;4:183–7.
24. Sharp NE, Aguayo P, Marx DJ, et al. Nursing preference of topical silver sulfadiazine versus collagenase ointment for treatment of partial thickness burns in children: survey follow-up of a prospective randomized trial. J Trauma Nurs 2014;21: 253–7.
25. Swaim SF, Lee AH. Topical wound medications - a review. J Am Vet Med Assoc 1987;190:1588–93.
26. Lee AH, Swaim SF, Yang ST, et al. Effects of gentamicin solution and cream on the healing of open wounds. Am J Vet Res 1984;45:1487–92.
27. Canapp SO Jr, Farese JP, Schultz GS, et al. The effect of topical tripeptide-copper complex on healing of ischemic open wounds. Vet Surg 2003;32:515–23.
28. Sierra-Garcia GD, Castro-Rios R, Gonzalez-Horta A, et al. Acemannan, an extracted polysaccharide from Aloe vera: a literature review. Nat Prod Commun 2014;9:1217–21.
29. Tanaka A, Nagate T, Matsuda H. Acceleration of wound healing by gelatin film dressings with epidermal growth factor. J Vet Med Sci 2005;67:909–13.
30. Carter CA, Jolly DG, Worden CE, et al. Platelet-rich plasma gel promotes differentiation and regeneration during equine wound healing. Exp Mol Pathol 2003; 74:244–55.
31. Tambella AM, Attili AR, Dini F, et al. Autologous platelet gel to treat chronic decubital ulcers: a randomized, blind controlled clinical trial in dogs. Vet Surg 2014;43: 726–33.
32. Monteiro SO, Lepage OM, Theoret CL. Effects of platelet-rich plasma on the repair of wounds on the distal aspect of the forelimb in horses. Am J Vet Res 2009;70:277–82.
33. Martinez-Zapata MJ, Marti-Carvajal AJ, Sola I, et al. Autologous platelet-rich plasma for treating chronic wounds. Cochrane Database Syst Rev 2012;(10):CD006899.
34. Ueno H, Mori T, Fujinaga T. Topical formulations and wound healing applications of chitosan. Adv Drug Deliv Rev 2001;52:105–15.
35. Senel S, McClure SJ. Potential applications of chitosan in veterinary medicine. Adv Drug Deliv Rev 2004;56:1467–80.
36. Shigemasa Y, Minami S. Applications of chitin and chitosan for biomaterials. Biotechnol Genet Eng Rev 1996;13:383–420.
37. Swaim SF, Gillette RL, Sartin EA, et al. Effects of a hydrolyzed collagen dressing on the healing of open wounds in dogs. Am J Vet Res 2000;61:1574–8.
38. Cooper R. Using honey to inhibit wound pathogens. Nurs Times 2008;104(46): 48–9.
39. Bell SG. The therapeutic use of honey. Neonatal Netw 2007;26:247–51.
40. Mathews KA, Binnington AG. Wound management using sugar. Compend Cont Educ Pract Vet 2002;24:41–50.
41. Chirife J, Scarmato G, Herszage L. Scientific basis for use of granulated sugar in treatment of infected wounds. Lancet 1982;1:560–1.
42. Morgan PW, Binnington AG, Miller CW, et al. The effect of occlusive and semi-occlusive dressings on the healing of acute full-thickness skin wounds on the forelimbs of dogs. Vet Surg 1994;23:494–502.

43. Ramsey DT, Pope ER, Wagnermann C, et al. Effects of 3 occlusive dressing materials on healing of full-thickness skin wounds in dogs. Am J Vet Res 1995; 56:941–9.

44. Lee AH, Swaim SF, Mcguire JA, et al. Effects of nonadherent dressing materials on the healing of open wounds in dogs. J Am Vet Med Assoc 1987;190:416–22.

45. Seaman S. Dressing selection in chronic wound management. J Am Podiatr Med Assoc 2002;92:24–33.

46. Lee WR, Tobias KM, Bemis DA, et al. In vitro efficacy of a polyhexamethylene biguanide-impregnated gauze dressing against bacteria found in veterinary patients. Vet Surg 2004;33:404–11.

47. Bowler PG, Jones SA, Walker M, et al. Microbicidal properties of a silver-containing hydrofiber dressing against a variety of burn wound pathogens. J Burn Care Rehabil 2004;25:192–6.

48. Jones SA, Bowler PG, Walker M, et al. Controlling wound bioburden with a novel silver-containing hydrofiber dressing. Wound Repair Regen 2004;12:288–94.

49. Kranke P, Bennett MH, Martyn-St James M, et al. Hyperbaric oxygen therapy for chronic wounds. Cochrane Database Syst Rev 2012;(4):CD004123.

50. Edwards ML. Hyperbaric oxygen therapy. Part 2: application in disease. J Vet Emerg Crit Care (San Antonio) 2010;20:289–97.

51. Camporesi EM. Side effects of hyperbaric oxygen therapy. Undersea Hyperb Med 2014;41:253–7.

52. Link KA, Koenig JB, Silveira A, et al. Effect of unfocused extracorporeal shock wave therapy on growth factor gene expression in wounds and intact skin of horses. Am J Vet Res 2013;74:324–32.

53. Morgan DD, McClure S, Yaeger MJ, et al. Effects of extracorporeal shock wave therapy on wounds of the distal portion of the limbs in horses. J Am Vet Med Assoc 2009;234:1154–61.

54. Haupt G, Chvapil M. Effect of shock waves on the healing of partial-thickness wounds in piglets. J Surg Res 1990;49:45–8.

55. Dymarek R, Halski T, Ptaszkowski K, et al. Extracorporeal shock wave therapy as an adjunct wound treatment: a systematic review of the literature. Ostomy Wound Manage 2014;60:26–39.

56. Rezende SB, Ribeiro MS, Nunez SC, et al. Effects of a single near-infrared laser treatment on cutaneous wound healing: biometrical and histological study in rats. J Photochem Photobiol B 2007;87:145–53.

57. Kawalec JS, Hetherington VJ, Pfennigwerth TC, et al. Effect of a diode laser on wound healing by using diabetic and nondiabetic mice. J Foot Ankle Surg 2004;43:214–20.

58. Woodruff LD, Bounkeo JM, Brannon WM, et al. The efficacy of laser therapy in wound repair: a meta-analysis of the literature. Photomed Laser Surg 2004;22:241–7.

59. Lucroy MD, Edwards BF, Madewell BR. Low-intensity laser light-induced closure of a chronic wound in a dog. Vet Surg 1999;28:292–5.

60. Lucas C, Criens-Poublon LJ, Cockrell CT, et al. Wound healing in cell studies and animal model experiments by low level laser therapy; were clinical studies justified? A systematic review. Lasers Med Sci 2002;17:110–34.

61. Millis DL, Gross Saunders D. Laser therapy in canine rehabilitation. In: Millis DL, Levine D, editors. Canine rehabilitation and physical therapy. 2nd edition. Philadelphia, PA: Elsevier; 2014. p. 359–80.

62. Kloth LC. Electrical stimulation for wound healing: a review of evidence from in vitro studies, animal experiments, and clinical trials. Int J Low Extrem Wounds 2005;4:23–44.

63. Bogie KM, Reger SI, Levine SP, et al. Electrical stimulation for pressure sore prevention and wound healing. Assist Technol 2000;12:50–66.
64. Belanger AY. Therapeutic electrophysical agents: evidence behind practice. 2nd edition. Philadelphia: Lippincott Williams & Wilkins; 2013.
65. Franek A, Polak A, Kucharzewski M. Modern application of high voltage stimulation for enhanced healing of venous crural ulceration. Med Eng Phys 2000;22: 647–55.
66. Houghton PE, Kincaid CB, Lovell M, et al. Effect of electrical stimulation on chronic leg ulcer size and appearance. Phys Ther 2003;83:17–28.
67. Peters EJ, Lavery LA, Armstrong DG, et al. Electric stimulation as an adjunct to heal diabetic foot ulcers: a randomized clinical trial. Arch Phys Med Rehabil 2001;82:721–5.
68. Leung MC, Ng GY, Yip KK. Effect of ultrasound on acute inflammation of transected medial collateral ligaments. Arch Phys Med Rehabil 2004;85:963–6.
69. Watson T. Ultrasound in contemporary physiotherapy practice. Ultrasonics 2008; 48:321–9.
70. Ramirez A, Schwane JA, McFarland C, et al. The effect of ultrasound on collagen synthesis and fibroblast proliferation in vitro. Med Sci Sports Exerc 1997;29: 326–32.
71. Nussbaum E. The influence of ultrasound on healing tissues. J Hand Ther 1998; 11:140–7.
72. Kavros SJ, Miller JL, Hanna SW. Treatment of ischemic wounds with noncontact, low-frequency ultrasound: the Mayo Clinic experience, 2004–2006. Adv Skin Wound Care 2007;20:221–6.
73. Kavros SJ, Schenck EC. Use of noncontact low-frequency ultrasound in the treatment of chronic foot and leg ulcerations: a 51-patient analysis. J Am Podiatr Med Assoc 2007;97:95–101.
74. Ennis WJ, Valdes W, Gainer M, et al. Evaluation of clinical effectiveness of MIST ultrasound therapy for the healing of chronic wounds. Adv Skin Wound Care 2006;19:437–46.

Current Concepts in Negative Pressure Wound Therapy

Lisa M. Howe, DVM, PhD

KEYWORDS

- Negative pressure wound therapy (NPWT) • Vacuum-assisted closure (VAC) • Dogs
- Cats • Wound care • Wounds

KEY POINTS

- Negative pressure wound therapy (NPWT) has been effective in the treatment of a wide range of complex wounds in human medicine, and its use in veterinary medicine is expanding.
- Patients treated with NPWT achieve wound closure quicker than patients treated with other traditional modalities.
- NPWT has been demonstrated to improve skin graft "take" compared with traditionally used bandaging techniques.
- Numerous mechanisms work together with NPWT to increase blood perfusion, speed up granulation tissue formation, and hasten wound contraction.
- As the number and variety of NPWT devices and materials increase, it is important to understand the different modes and components of NPWT devices and how to select materials appropriately based on the selected mode of operation.

INTRODUCTION

Management of traumatic and surgical wounds is a frequent event in small animal veterinary practice. Dogs and cats possess an uncanny ability to suffer injury in the most inconceivable ways, and these injuries, as well as more common injuries, often require wound care for several days before the wound environment is suitable for closure. In addition, surgical wound infections occur and require wound care until the infection has cleared and closure, when needed, is appropriate.

Veterinarians regularly search for materials and methods of wound management that improve wound environment, speed up wound healing, provide comfort for the

The author has nothing to disclose.
Department of Small Animal Clinical Sciences, College of Veterinary Medicine and Biomedical Sciences, Texas A&M University, College Station, TX 77843-4474, USA
E-mail address: lhowe@cvm.tamu.edu

vetsmall.theclinics.com

patient during healing, and minimize the frequency of sedation or anesthesia for wound care and bandage changes. Practitioners also look for wound healing strategies that are inexpensive for their clients and minimally labor intensive for themselves and their technical staff.

One wound healing strategy that addresses many of these concerns is NPWT, also referred to as vacuum-assisted closure (VAC) or topical negative (wound) therapy or pressure. NPWT has been used extensively in human medicine as an advanced wound healing strategy for more than a decade, and veterinarians are using the technique as well. NPWT is reported to enhance wound environment to the degree that granulation tissue forms more quickly and wounds heal in shorter times than with traditional or wet-to-dry bandaging.

This article discusses the theory and mechanism of action of NPWT, describes the indications (and contraindications) for NPWT, describes the technique for application of the NPWT bandage and device, discusses the advantages and disadvantages of NPWT, and explores some of the new techniques and future directions of NPWT in human medicine that may prove useful for the veterinary patient.

ORIGIN AND DESCRIPTION OF NEGATIVE PRESSURE WOUND THERAPY

Origins of the use of medical vacuum dates back thousands of years, but the use of medical vacuum in modern times dates back only about 20 years. Ancient people used animal horns, bamboo canes, and other items to create a vacuum using their mouths and then seal the hole with a plug of wax or other material held in their mouths to maintain the vacuum.[1] Numerous modifications of these devices were developed and used through the early 1900s.[2–4] These devices were thought to result in venous hyperemia for treatment of suppurative inflammatory diseases. However, many of these vacuum devices fell into disfavor until about the end of the twentieth century.

NPWT began to come into widespread use in human medicine in 1997 after the publication of 2 articles describing VAC.[5,6] Since then, the use of NPWT has become commonplace in human hospital settings. The use of NPWT has become more widespread in veterinary medicine in recent years, although the scientific literature in veterinary species is sparse. There are several reports describing the use of NPWT in individual cats,[7,8] horses,[9] and dogs,[10] as well as a few exotic animal species.[11–13] There are also a case series[14] and controlled experimental studies.[15,16]

NPWT involves the use of a vacuum, or suction, applied to an open wound that has been covered with porous foam that is then covered by an adherent, occlusive sheet of plastic bandage material to achieve an airtight seal. Controlled negative (subatmospheric) pressure is applied to the wound, pulling exudates and effusions through the foam and into a reservoir and bathing the wound in tissue fluids from inside to outside to provide a healthy wound environment without maceration.

PROPOSED MECHANISMS OF ACTION OF NEGATIVE PRESSURE WOUND THERAPY

Numerous mechanisms of action have been proposed for the clinical benefits seen with NPWT, many of which work together to improve the wound environment and optimize the healing process (**Box 1**).

Several studies have demonstrated increased perfusion to wounded tissue during NPWT.[5,17–20] In the landmark study by Morykwas and colleagues,[5] blood flow to the wounds (as measured by Doppler ultrasonography) increased 4-fold when 125 mm Hg negative pressure was applied to the wounds and survival of random pattern flaps increased by 21% compared with controls. Other studies have shown similar results.[17–20] In addition to the effect of the actual negative pressure on blood

---

Box 1
Proposed mechanisms of action of NPWT

- Increased perfusion
- Enhanced formation of granulation tissue
- Reduced bacterial levels*
- Removal of exudate
- Reduction of tissue edema
- Decreased proinflammatory cytokines
- Decreased proteases

*Literature results are mixed relative to this mechanism of action.

---

flow, other mechanisms may be at work. Nitric oxide (NO) has been demonstrated to play a role in the circulatory change seen in wounds treated with NPWT.[21] In the NO study, an NO synthase inhibitor (N^G-nitro-L-arginine methyl ester [L-NAME]) was administered and the inhibitor almost completely blocked the effect of NPWT in increasing the wound bed blood flow. It has also been found that the vascular response seen with NPWT is related to the physical presence of polyurethane foam.[22] In that study, wounds exposed to uncompressed and compressed foam (without NPWT), or to standard NPWT, showed a 2-fold increase in vascularity compared with the occlusive dressing (no foam) with NPWT.

Good blood perfusion to a wound is needed to deliver oxygen and nutrients, as well as cells and growth factors, to the injured tissue. In addition, with increased perfusion there is increased delivery of antimicrobials to the wound in a patient receiving systemic antimicrobials.[23] Increased blood perfusion also benefits a wound by removing free radicals, carbon dioxide, and waste products.[24]

The blood flow in different areas of the wound is such that some areas of the wound are hyperperfused and some areas are hypoperfused[18–22,25]; this is thought to be due to differing forces acting on the tissues in the superficial and deep portions of the wound (**Fig. 1**). Macrodeformations are those tissue deformations that result from the centripetal pulling of the wound edges caused by the NPWT.[15,22,24,26,27] Effects of these macrodeformations differ depending on tissue depth of the wound.[24,26,27] The superficial portion of the wound is subjected to compressive forces, which results in hypoperfusion. Deep portions of the wound are subjected to traction forces. This traction results in widening of the blood vessels leading to hyperperfusion. The superficial hypoperfusion and hypoxia results in a vascular endothelial growth factor gradient that promotes sprouting angiogenesis. The deep hyperperfusion increases nutrient and oxygen delivery. Hyperperfusion has also been documented at distances of 2.5 cm from the wound edges.[20,25]

Microdeformations are caused by the interaction between the foam and the surface of the wound in contact with the foam.[20,25,26] Microdeformations have also been demonstrated to be important factors in the efficacy of NPWT in cellular proliferation and increased granulation tissue production through the action of NPWT on myofibroblasts. Mechanical stress on the tissues by NPWT seems to activate transforming growth factor 1, which is critical for the vacuum-induced myofibroblast differentiation.[20,25,26] In addition, myofibroblasts are important in vessel translocation (looping angiogenesis), which results in the neovascularization seen during wound healing and wound contraction.[20,25,26]

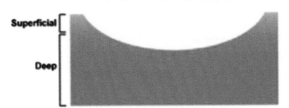

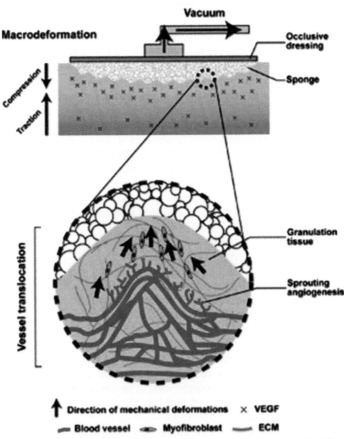

Fig. 1. Mechanisms of action of NPWT, including macrodeformations (*middle portion of figure*) and microdeformations (*bottom of figure*). Macrodeformations are tissue deformations caused by the centripetal forces pulling the wound margins. Microdeformations are tissue deformations caused by foam and wound dressing interactions. ECM, extracellular matrix; VEGF, vascular endothelial growth factor. (*From* Daigle P, Despatis MA, Grenier G. How mechanical deformations contribute to the effectiveness of negative-pressure wound therapy. Wound Repair Regen 2013;21:499; with permission.)

Reduced bacterial burden in the wound has been proposed as a mechanism that leads to improved wound healing with NPWT, a point advertised to do such by some manufacturers of NPWT supplies. However, results on this issue have been mixed.[28-34] An early report found a reduction in bacterial loads with NPWT usage in pig wounds inoculated with *Staphylococcus epidermidis* and *Staphylococcus aureus*.[5] Other clinical studies have not documented a decrease in wound bacterial loads,[28,31,32] and some have shown an increase.[33,34] Additional research is needed to determine the effects of NPWT on bacterial burden in the wound itself (rather than on the foam or gauze used as packing material in the wound). Regardless of whether bioburden is decreased, wound healing with NPWT seems to progress extremely quickly. It seems reasonable to speculate that wound bioburden is affected by wound fluid removal from infected wounds. Gauze impregnated with polyhexamethylene biguanide reduces bacterial load in wounds.[35] Other pathogen-binding materials would also be expected to have similar results.

NPWT results in active drainage of wound exudates and, as such, is an effective tool for decreasing edema.[6,24,26,36,37] The removal of excess interstitial fluid results in decreased interstitial pressure and decrease in edema.[5,27,36] The effectiveness of fluid removal depends on direct contact between the wound bed and the filler material, the negative pressure applied to the wound, and the type of material used as a filler. Fluid removal from the wound was more effective with foam and pathogen-binding mesh than with gauze at pressures of -80 and -120 mm Hg.[25] Perhaps healing would be somewhat slower in wounds in which there is less effective fluid removal and nonantimicrobial gauze is used.

Fluid removal with NPWT is also beneficial because it alters the fluid composition in the wound.[38-41] Fluid removal decreases the levels of cytokines, metalloproteinases, plasmin, thrombin, elastase, and other proteolytic enzymes, which negatively affect wound healing.[15,24] This change in fluid composition has been demonstrated in several studies examining the effects of NPWT on levels of metalloproteinases and cytokines.[42-44] Removal of these proinflammatory cytokines and proteases improves wound healing.[6,43-45]

INDICATIONS/CONTRAINDICATIONS

There are numerous indications for NPWT in veterinary medicine (**Box 2**). The primary indication includes wounds of all types and configurations.[5-9,15,45] NPWT is also used with skin grafts and flaps and is reported to result in improved graft take (the author's anecdotal experience supports this observation).[14,16] Other indications in human medicine that are used rarely in veterinary medicine thus far include NPWT for open abdomen management,[46-51] closed incisional management,[52-54] and installation NPWT (see later discussion).[55-59] These techniques may become more commonplace in veterinary medicine in the future.

Some contraindications for NPWT should be kept in mind when selecting patients for this treatment modality (see **Box 2**). NPWT should not be used in the presence of any local malignancy, because it is reported to have led to tumor recurrence in a human and could potentially lead to spread of the tumor throughout the wound bed.[60]

Untreated osteomyelitis is also considered a contraindication for NPWT, as bone fragments could dislodge and puncture the plastic sheet and result in loss of suction or tissue damage if sharp edges are present.[26] Such cases should be thoroughly surgically debrided of all necrotic and nonviable tissue before the initiation of NPWT.[6,26] Necrotic bone fragments in cases of osteomyelitis can become covered with granulation tissue and lead to sequestration.[7] NPWT should not be used over exposed vessels,

---

Box 2
Indications and contraindications of NPWT

Indications

- Acute traumatic wounds
- Chronic wounds
- Dehisced wounds
- Burns
- Ulcers
- Skin grafts
- Skin flaps
- Closed surgical wounds
- Open abdomens

Contraindications

- Remaining tumor in a wound bed
- Undebrided osteomyelitis
- Exposed vessels, nerves, tendons, or ligaments
- Patients with bleeding or coagulation disorders
- Patients receiving anticoagulants that cannot be carefully monitored
- Active bleeding or over unsutured hemostatic agents
- Unprotected organs or anastatomotic sites
- Eschar over necrotic tissue unless removed
- Unexplored fistulae
- Unexplored wounds that could connect with the chest or abdomen

---

tendons, ligaments, and nerves because damage could occur and severe hemorrhage could result if NPWT is placed over arteries or veins.[26] Unprotected organs or anastomotic sites are also contraindications for use of NPWT, unless they can be well covered by a nonadherent polyethylene sheet or other suitable nonadherent material placed over viscera to protect from subatmospheric pressure before initiation of NPWT.[26]

NPWT should not be used in patients with bleeding and coagulation disorders (or those receiving anticoagulants) or in patients in which unsutured hemostatic agents have been placed in a wound because the agents could dislodge and result in severe hemorrhage. The presence of an eschar over necrotic tissue is a contraindication until the eschar and necrotic tissue are completely removed.[26] The use of NPWT is also contraindicated in unexplored fistulae or wounds that could have unseen connections with the chest or abdomen.

SELECTION OF MATERIALS

There are several companies offering NPWT equipment and supplies. These companies often have prepackaged kits that contain all the supplies needed for an individual patient, which is a great convenience. The selection of these kits often depends on the type of NPWT therapy being used (**Fig. 2**). Vacuum may be applied with or without

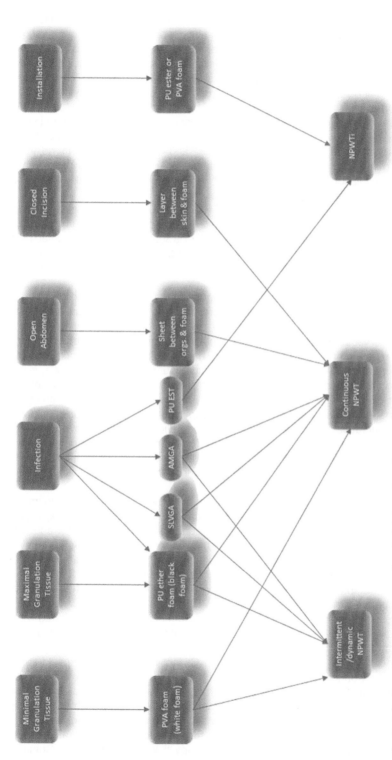

Fig. 2. Selection of NPWT therapy and materials based on tissue application, environment, and desired action on tissue. AMGA, antimicrobial gauze; EST, ester; NPWT, installation NPWT; PU, polyurethane; PVA, polyvinyl alcohol; SLVPU, silver-impregnated polyurethane.

installation of fluids into the wound. If the wound is both to be lavaged and to receive NPWT (NPWT instill [NPWTi]), then different kits containing different configurations of vacuum pads and foam type should be selected. Although veterinary usage of NPWTi has not been reported, it has been reported to have advantages for certain human wounds. Vacuum pumps that have both standard NPWT and NPWTi functions in the same machine (V.A.C. Ulta Negative Pressure Wound Therapy System, KCI, Inc, San Antonio, TX, USA) are available.

Installation therapy has been recommended for contaminated and infected wounds that could benefit from lavage therapy coupled with NPWT.[61] With installation therapy, topical solutions (eg, antiseptics, cleansers, and antimicrobials) can be instilled directly to the wound bed in a controlled fashion. Such therapy has been shown to improve granulation tissue production.[56–60] Installation NPWT has also been shown to have possible benefit in noncontaminated wounds.[57,62,63]

With NPWTi, retrograde installation of topical solutions occurs into the sealed wound bed using an additional tubing system while the vacuum pump is paused, causing the foam to become soaked. The wound is soaked for a user-selected period. During the soak time, the topical solution is in contact with the foam and wound surface. Once the soak time is completed, negative pressure resumes and the remaining fluid is removed from the foam.

NPWT can also have differing suction modes that are user selected on some vacuum pumps (see **Fig. 2**).[59] Two modes are available, continuous and intermittent. With continuous suction, the clinician-set pressure is constant during therapy as long as the vacuum pump remains on (and the airtight seal is intact). This suction mode is most commonly used in veterinary medicine, and it is the mode used in the author's hospital. One type of noncontinuous pressure is intermittent NPWT, in which a set negative pressure is alternated with no pressure for programmed periods. The second type of noncontinuous NPWT is dynamic, or variable, NPWT. With dynamic NPWT, negative pressure transitions between high and low pressures follow programmed increase and decrease times. Some studies suggest improved granulation tissue production with both intermittent and dynamic NPWT compared with that observed with continuous NPWT,[5,64,65] although one study did not.[66] Intermittent suction causes more pain than continuous suction in human patients, especially with higher pressures.[17,67,68]

Different types of foam may also be selected. The commonly used foam types include polyurethane (PU) foam (black foam; can be PU ether or ester), polyvinylalcohol foam (white foam), antimicrobial-impregnated gauze or mesh, and silver-impregnated black foam (see **Fig. 2**). At the author's institution, before kits were readily available, sterilized thick black speaker foam, red rubber catheters, appropriate connectors and canisters, and wall or portable suction units for NPWT were used. This setup resulted in subjectively greatly improved granulation tissue production compared with standard wet-to-dry bandages with far fewer bandage changes. It was subjectively more cumbersome to place and maintain NPWT compared with the kits that are currently used. In addition, accuracy of suction pressure selected was not as precise with the homemade device.

Black foam (V.A.C. GranuFoam Dressing, KCI, Inc) is probably used most frequently in veterinary wounds, and it is indicated for most veterinary applications in small animals (see **Fig. 2**). Both ether and ester forms of black foam have similarly sized reticulated open cells (400–600 µm); however, the ether form is slightly more hydrophobic.[45] Because of this, the ether form (V.A.C. GranuFoam Dressing) is recommended for use with standard NPWT, whereas the ester form (V.A.C. VeraFlo Dressing, KCI, Inc) is recommended for installation therapy.[45] White foam (V.A.C. GranuFoam

WhiteFoam Dressing, KCI, Inc) has much smaller open cells that stimulate less granulation tissue; therefore, this foam should probably not be selected for use with deep wounds that need heavy granulation tissue formation to fill a cavity.[6,69]

Antimicrobial-impregnated medical gauze sponge (Kerlix AMD, Covidien, Mansfield, MA, USA) has been used frequently in human medicine, but its use in veterinary medicine has not been reported.[17,67,69–72] It seems to be particularly useful because of its ease of application and moldability. More fluid is retained in the wound with gauze than with foam or antimicrobial-impregnated mesh, despite the fact that pressure transduction within the wound is similar to that for foam or mesh.[25,38] Wound contraction is less than that seen with foam.[25,69,73,74]

Antimicrobial-impregnated mesh (Cutimed Sorbact, BSN Medical, Inc, Charlotte, NC, USA) has been used for prevention and treatment of acute traumatic, postsurgical, and hard-to-heal wounds and burns.[25] It has been used with NPWT and was found to provide similar pressure transduction throughout the wound as black foam and antimicrobial gauze, but wound contraction for antimicrobial mesh was less than that of foam.[25] Silver-impregnated black foam (V.A.C. GranuFoam Silver Dressing, KCI, Inc) contains elemental silver (10%) as a sustained release formulation, and its use in infected wounds as an adjunct to standard treatment regimens is suggested.[45,69,75–78] It cannot be used with installation therapy because any topical agent or solution may have an adverse reaction with silver and compromise the effectiveness of the dressing.[45]

TECHNIQUE/PROCEDURE

The technique of placement and use of NPWT involves several consistent steps regardless of wound location (**Fig. 3**). The steps include wound preparation, application of foam or other wound filler and dressing, application of vacuum pad device, attachment of the NPWT unit, and close monitoring of the NPWT for loss of suction or other problems.

Complete wound preparation and exploration should occur before beginning NPWT. The presence of wound debris or necrotic tissue adversely affects NPWT wound healing. As noted earlier, if an eschar is present, it must be removed along with any necrotic tissue present under the eschar.

When the foam (or other wound filler material) is placed, one must completely fill the wound cavity to ensure that the vacuum over the wound surface works optimally. To prevent inadvertent foreign body retention, the number of pieces of foam placed in the wound should be counted and recorded in the medical record. It is important to be careful that the filler material does not overlap the skin edge as maceration and skin damage may occur.

A Tegaderm dressing (Tegaderm Film, 3M, 3M Center, St Paul, MN, USA), or other self-adhering occlusive plastic sheeting, is applied over the foam and secured to the skin. Although the instructions supplied with the kit recommend that the Tegaderm overlap the skin edges by 3 to 5 cm, the author prefers to overlap the skin edges by at least 4 to 6 cm, if the location of the wound allows. It is preferable to have as few wrinkles in the Tegaderm as possible during the application process, and the Tegaderm must be securely affixed to the skin. If a single large Tegaderm is too difficult to apply, it may be cut into smaller pieces and applied to the wound, being certain to overlap sufficiently the previously placed section of Tegaderm.

When cutting the hole in the Tegaderm dressing to permit placement of the self-adhering vacuum pad, the hole should not be cut too small such that it impedes the vacuum pull. Likewise, the vacuum pad through which suction is pulled must not

Wound Preparation
- Wide clip and scrub of wound edges to permit sufficient area to affix drapes
- Copious lavage with lavage solution of choice and wound debridement
- Dry edges of skin with sterile towel so that drapes will adhere appropriately
- Be certain no vessels or nerves are exposed.

Apply Foam
- Cut foam to the appropriate size and insert into the wound
- Ensure that all tunnels and crevices have been examined and packed with foam
- Record how many foam pieces were placed into wound
- Allow no foam to overlap skin edges

Apply Dressing
- Apply a Tegaderm dressing such that the foam is covered with an additional 4-6 cm border covering all periwound skin edges
- The Tegaderm dressing may be cut into smaller pieces if needed to facilitate complete coverage of the wound and ease of handling

Apply Vacuum Pad
- Select a location over the foam (often the center) for the pad to be placed
- Grasp the Tegaderm drape at this location and pinch it upward
- Cut a 2.5-cm hole through the Tegaderm dressing and stick pad in place
- Apply another small piece of Tegaderm to cover pad and secure it

Attach NPWT Unit
- Attach vacuum pad tubing to unit tubing
- Be sure clamps on both tubes are open
- Select appropriate settings and turn on the power to the NPWT device
- Ensure integrity of the seal – vacuum and dressing should collapse

Monitor
- Preferably check system every 2 hours for loss of suction
- Frequently record volume and character of fluid collected in canister and empty
- Patient checks to ascertain hydration status, protein levels, and comfort
- Change bandage at least every 3 days

Fig. 3. Steps involved in NPWT application. The first 3 arrows and associated text boxes represent the steps of wound preparation and foam and dressing application, whereas the second set of 3 arrows and associated text boxes represent the portion of the procedure related to the application of the suction pads and devices.

overlap the skin edges, as this potentially affects the vacuum pressure on the wound and also results in tissue damage to the skin. Although not recommended by the manufacturer, the author routinely applies a small piece of Tegaderm over the top of the vacuum pad (that is affixed to the foam) and tubing so the pad cannot inadvertently become dislodged and separated from the foam.

After all tubing has been correctly attached and clamps opened, the unit is ready to start. The mode of operation (continuous, intermittent, dynamic, or installation) must be set along with the appropriate vacuum pressure. Pressures typically have been set at −125 mm Hg for most utilizations and −75 to −80 mm Hg for use with skin grafts. Studies from the literature suggest, however, that pressures of −75 to −100 mm Hg may be more appropriate for optimal wound healing.[20,64,79] After the machine variables have been set, the vacuum unit is started. The foam and top dressing must be observed to ensure that the foam contracts down and that there are no leaks in the NPWT system. Once it has been ascertained that there are no leaks, monitoring of the system should begin.

CARE AND MONITORING OF NEGATIVE PRESSURE WOUND THERAPY

Appropriate care and monitoring of the NPWT is extremely important in achieving a positive effect on wound healing rate and quality (see **Fig. 3**). Check the system frequently for any evidence of suction loss. Ideally, the system should be monitored at least every 2 hours, because it is recommended that the foam and dressing be changed and the wound be flushed after 2 hours of suction loss. Additional dressing changes would result in increased labor and costs. Should suction loss occur, examine the system to determine the location of suction loss, correct the cause of suction loss (if <2 hours), and restart the unit. Many vacuum pumps have seal check leak detectors with audio alarms that signal if a leak is detected. Such a feature can be of great assistance in a busy practice.

The character and volume of the fluid being suctioned from the wound need to be monitored to determine the effectiveness of NPWT in controlling infection and to determine that drainage volume is declining. The canister also needs to be emptied or changed as it approaches its maximum capacity and the volume recorded.

Dressings may be left in place for up to 3 days before changing, although the author often performs dressing changes after 48 hours.[15,16] Changing the bandage at 48-hour intervals helps avoid granulation tissue growth into the sponge, as well as allows more frequent checking of the wound bed. The wound can be assessed at each bandage change, paying particular attention to the health and amount of granulation tissue. The degree of contraction should be assessed and recorded. Once a healthy bed of granulation tissue has formed, NPWT should be discontinued and closure or reconstruction performed.

The patient should also be intermittently monitored to ensure protein levels and hydration status are maintained, particularly with large heavily exuding wounds or open abdomens, although this seems to be a rare problem in humans.[6] During bandage changes of large wounds, sedation may be needed. The patient's pain score should be monitored frequently and appropriate analgesia administered. Devices (eg, e-collars, side braces) to prevent the patient from disturbing the NPWT should be placed.

COMPLICATIONS

Complications may occur with NPWT; however, most are preventable through attention to detail and vigilant monitoring (**Box 3**).[45,80] Loss of suction is probably one of the most common problems associated with NPWT. Vigilant monitoring and inspection of the bandage and tubing help prevent this problem, as does protection of materials from the patient.

If vessels are not covered with tissue, the suction can cause erosion of the vessels and result in significant hemorrhage.[6,45] If this occurs, the NPWT must be stopped immediately, hemorrhage controlled, and vessels covered before reimplementing NPWT or switching to a different bandaging system.

As previously noted, the presence of devitalized bone in a patient with fracture or osteomyelitis undergoing NPWT can result in coverage of the devitalized bone by granulation tissue and subsequent sequestration.[6,45] This situation has been reported

---

Box 3
Complications that may occur in small animal patients undergoing NPWT

- Loss of suction
- Erosion of vessels
- Dislodging of hemostatic agents
- Granulation tissue coverage of devitalized tissue; bony sequester
- Lack of response to therapy
- Pain
- Enteric fistula*

*Complication has not been reported in veterinary medicine but has potential to occur as more laparostomy NPWT is used.

---

in the human literature, but it illustrates the importance of careful debridement of necrotic tissue and devitalized bone in veterinary osteomyelitic patients before implementing NPWT.

Less frequent complications reported in the human literature include nonresponse to NPWT, skin erosion, and skin maceration. Rarely patients have been found to be unresponsive to NPWT, but insufficient wound debridement or failure to maintain NPWT for a sufficient length of time may have contributed to some of the reports.[6,45] Erosion of the skin from the vacuum tubing passing over the skin has been reported.[6] This report cites patients lying on their tubes, an event possible in nonambulatory veterinary patients. There exist sporadic reports of maceration of skin adjacent to the wound if foam or other cavity filler material overlap the skin edge, so care should be used in veterinary patients to avoid this.[6] Enteric fistulae have been reported in humans undergoing open-abdomen NPWT.[6,81,82]

Pain is commonly identified as a complication of NPWT in human patients, and in some patients pain is so severe that it results in discontinuation of the therapy.[6,64,69,83] Pain occurs most frequently when the vacuum unit is turned on and begins to pull a vacuum and typically subsides by 20 to 30 minutes.[6] Because typically veterinary patients receiving NPWT are heavily sedated during bandage placement and initiation of suction, the only time that the author has observed unsedated patients having vacuum restarted is after suction is lost. Overt discomfort or pain was not observed, but such patients are treated with analgesics. If there is ingrowth of granulation tissue into the sponge, dogs act painful as the sponge is being removed. Patient pain should be well controlled not only as part of a good patient care protocol but also to avoid stress in the patient.

ADVANTAGES AND DISADVANTAGES OF NEGATIVE PRESSURE WOUND THERAPY

Advantages and disadvantages of NPWT (**Box 4**) likely vary depending on the differing types of veterinary practices. Some practices are well suited for NPWT and can readily add this technology to wound management treatment options, whereas in other practices disadvantages may outweigh advantages. NPWT should probably not be used in practices that have no overnight monitoring of patients or a nearby 24-hour emergency clinic for overnight monitoring.

For practices that can provide NPWT, the therapeutic benefits outweigh the disadvantages. Those advantages include increased rate of healing, decreased labor (assuming suction loss can be avoided), and likely decreased client expense. The

> **Box 4**
> **Advantages and disadvantages of NPWT**
>
> Advantages
> - Improved wound healing
> - Early mobility
> - Possible earlier release from the hospital
> - Decreased labor
> - Possible cost savings to the client
> - Sets practice apart
> - Easy to learn technique
>
> Disadvantages
> - Some practices may not be well suited for NPWT
> - Initial equipment costs
> - Increased inventory
> - Must learn new technique

primary disadvantage of NPWT is the initial equipment expense and the learning curve (albeit steep) associated with NPWT.

OUTCOMES

In both anecdotal reports and the scientific literature, it is evident that NPWT offers great benefit for the patient in terms of speed of wound healing, such as the speed and improvement in vascularity, decreased edema, increased rate of granulation tissue formation, increased rate of wound contraction, potential decrease in bioburden, decreased bandage size and thickness (in most patients) that encourage early mobility, and potential shortened hospitalization.

FUTURE CONSIDERATIONS

In addition to installation NPWT, there are several interesting developments in the human medical field that likely have applicability to veterinary patients. Laparostomy NPWT, or open-abdomen NPWT, has been used successfully in human patients with septic peritonitis and has also been reported in veterinary medicine.[46,47,49,50,84,85] With laparostomy NPWT in humans, a special foam for abdominal usage (ABThera Open Abdomen Negative Pressure Therapy, KCI, Inc) is attached to visceral protective sheeting and inserted into the abdomen, making certain that the foam fingers are slid along the sides of the inner abdominal walls and rest deeply into the dorsal recesses of the abdominal cavity. The special usage foam is covered with a Tegaderm sheet and attached to the vacuum unit in a standard manner. In dogs and cats, homemade devices have been used to drain the abdomen. The caudal aspect of the abdomen is closed, whereas the cranial half is loosely closed, leaving a gap between the edges of the body wall, subcutaneous tissue, and skin. The foam is laid external to the loose body wall closure, a red-rubber catheter is inserted into the middle of the foam and attached to the suction canister, and the foam is covered using a Tegaderm dressing. In some instances, additional bandaging materials were placed over the Tegaderm dressing. Mortality rates reported in the veterinary literature were approximately 50% using this technique. This mortality rate is similar or higher than most of those reported for open abdominal drainage (33%–48%) or closed suction drains (30%) in dogs and cats.[86–90]

NPWT has become useful in human medicine for closed surgical incisions.[53,54,91–93] Patients selected for this therapy are typically orthopedic (fractures or total joint replacements) or sternotomy patients that are at high risk for incisional healing issues or dehiscence. It has been calculated that when NPWT has been applied over a surgically closed incision, the force required to disrupt the incision increases by 50% in a model of freshly incised skin.[94] The NPWT is applied immediately postoperatively, and a nonadherent layer is placed between the foam dressing and the skin to prevent possible skin maceration. Alternatively, a dressing that is designed for this purpose and is skin friendly (Prevena Incision Management System, KCI, Inc) may be used and can be attached to a standard pump or a portable, single-use device.

Single-use, portable pumps that are preset to −80 mm Hg are a recent new development in human medicine.[94–96] The life span of these devices is typically 1 week. Although patients return for dressing changes and wound checks, the cost savings is remarkable and patients are often able to return to their normal lifestyle (including work), thus improving patient outlook, appetite, stress levels, and overall well-being. These devices may prove useful to select veterinary patients and could potentially be secured to dogs' bodies with a vest similar to that used to attach Holter monitors to veterinary patients.

The use of stem cells and scaffolds combined with NPWT may offer new treatment options for complex wounds. Such therapy has been examined for use in human medicine, and it may prove useful in both human and veterinary medicine in the future.[26] As newer, improved equipment and increased applications become available for NPWT in human medicine, veterinary patients of all sizes may benefit by having more options for complex wound management.

SUMMARY

- NPWT has been effective in the treatment of a wide range of complex wounds in human medicine, and its use in veterinary medicine is increasing.
- Patients treated with NPWT achieve wound closure quicker than patients treated with other traditional modalities.
- NPWT has been demonstrated to improve skin graft take compared with traditionally used bandaging techniques.
- Numerous mechanisms work together with NPWT to increase blood perfusion, speed up granulation tissue formation, and hasten contraction of wounds.
- As the number and variety of NPWT devices and materials increase, it is important to understand the different modes and components of NPWT devices and how to select materials appropriately based on the selected mode of operation.
- Before purchase of equipment and use of NPWT, it is important to understand the indications and contraindications, as well as the advantages and disadvantages of NPWT for each patient and practice situation.

REFERENCES

1. Larichev A. At the beginning of vacuum therapy: from the blood-sucking cups to the Bier-Klapp method. Neg Press Wound Ther 2014;1:5–9.
2. Murray Y. On the local and general influence on body, of increased and diminished atmospheric pressure. Lancet 1835;3:909–17.

3. Heaton G. Note on the drainage of large cavities after surgical operation. Br Med J 1898;1:207–8.
4. Chaffin RC. Surgical drainage. Am J Surg 1934;24:100–4.
5. Morykwas MJ, Argenta LC, Shelton-Brown EI, et al. Vacuum-assisted closure: a new method for wound control and treatment: animal studies and basic foundation. Ann Plast Surg 1997;38:553–62.
6. Argenta LC, Morykwas MJ. Vacuum-assisted closure: a new method for wound control and treatment: clinical experience. Ann Plast Surg 1997;38:563–77.
7. Guille AE, Tseng LW, Orsher RJ. Use of vacuum-assisted closure for management of a large skin wound in a cat. J Am Vet Med Assoc 2007;230:1669–73.
8. Owen L, Hotston-Moore A, Holt P. Vacuum-assisted wound closure following urine-induced skin and thigh muscle necrosis in a cat. Vet Comp Orthop Traumatol 2009;22:417–21.
9. Gemeinhardt KD, Molnar JA. Vacuum-assisted closure for management of a traumatic neck wound in a horse. Equine Vet Educ 2005;17:27–33.
10. Mullally C, Carey K, Seshadri R. Use of a nanocrystalline silver dressing and vacuum-assisted closure in a severely burned dog. J Vet Emerg Crit Care 2010;20:456–63.
11. LaFortune M, Fleming GJ, Wheeler JL, et al. Wound management in a juvenile tiger (Panthera tigris) with vacuum-assisted closure (V.A.C.) therapy. J Zoo Wildl Med 2007;38:341–4.
12. Adkesson MJ, Travis EK, Weber MA, et al. Vacuum-assisted closure for treatment of a deep shell abscess and osteomyelitis in a tortoise. J Am Vet Med Assoc 2007;231:1249–54.
13. Harrison TM, Stanley BJ, Sikarski JG, et al. Surgical amputation of a digit and vacuum-assisted closure (V.A.C.) for management in a case of osteomyelitis and wound care in an eastern black rhinoceros (Diceros bicornis michaeli). J Zoo Wildl Med 2011;42:317–21.
14. Ben-Amotz R, Lanz OI, Miller JM, et al. The use of vacuum-assisted closure therapy for treatment of distal extremity wounds in 15 dogs. Vet Surg 2007;36:684–90.
15. Demaria M, Stanley BJ, Hauptman JG, et al. Effects of negative pressure wound therapy on healing of open wounds in dogs. Vet Surg 2011;40:658–69.
16. Stanley BJ, Pitt KA, Weder CD, et al. Effects of negative pressure wound therapy on the healing of free full-thickness skin grafts in dogs. Vet Surg 2013;42:511–22.
17. Timmers MS, Le Cessie S, Banwell P, et al. The effects of varying degrees of pressure delivered by negative-pressure wound therapy on skin perfusion. Ann Plast Surg 2005;55:665–71.
18. Wackenfors A, Gustafsson R, Sjogren J, et al. Blood flow responses in the peristernal thoracic wall during vacuum-assisted closure therapy. Ann Thorac Surg 2005;79:1724–30.
19. Wackenfors A, Sjogren J, Gustafsson R, et al. Effects of vacuum-assisted closure therapy on inguinal wound edge microvascular blood flow. Wound Repair Regen 2004;12:600–6.
20. Borgquist O, Ingemansson R, Malmsjo M. Wound edge microvascular blood flow during negative-pressure wound therapy: examining the effects of pressures from -10 to -175 mm Hg. Plast Reconstr Surg 2010;125:502–9.
21. Sano H, Ichioka S. Involvement of nitric oxide in the wound bed microcirculatory change during negative pressure wound therapy. Int Wound J 2013. http://dx.doi.org/10.1111/iwj.12121.
22. Scherer SS, Pietramaggiori G, Mathews JC, et al. The mechanism of action of the vacuum-assisted closure device. Plast Reconstr Surg 2008;122:786–97.

23. Cross SE, Thompson MJ, Roberts MS. Distribution of systemically administered ampicillin, benzylpenicillin, and flucloxacillin in excisional wounds in diabetic and normal rats and effects of local topical vasodilator treatment. Antimicrob Agents Chemother 1996;40:1703–10.

24. Hunter J, Teot L, Horch R, et al. Evidence-based medicine: vacuum-assisted closure in wound care management. Int Wound J 2007;4:256–69.

25. Malmsjo M, langemannson R, Lindstedt S, et al. Comparison of bacteria and fungus-binding mesh, foam, and gauze as fillers in negative pressure wound therapy – pressure transduction, wound edge contraction, microvascular blood flow and fluid retention. Int Wound J 2013;10:597–605.

26. Orgill DP, Bayer LR. Negative pressure wound therapy: past, present and future. Int Wound J 2013;10(Suppl 1):15–9.

27. Daigle P, Despatis MA, Grenier G. How mechanical deformations contribute to the effectiveness of negative-pressure wound therapy. Wound Repair Regen 2013;21:498–502.

28. Anesater E, Roupe KM, Robertsson P, et al. The influence on wound contraction and fluid evacuation of a rigid disc inserted to protect exposed organs during negative pressure wound therapy. Int Wound J 2011;8:393–9.

29. Orgill DP, Manders EK, Sumpio BE, et al. The mechanisms of action of vacuum assisted closure: more to learn. Surgery 2009;146:40–51.

30. Chester DL, Waters R. Adverse alteration of wound flora with topical negative-pressure therapy: a case report. Br J Plast Surg 2002;55:510–1.

31. Mous CM, Vos MC, van den Bemd GJ, et al. Bacterial load in relation to vacuum-assisted closure wound therapy: a prospective randomized trial. Wound Repair Regen 2004;12:11–7.

32. Khashram M, Huggan P, Ikram R, et al. Effect of TNP on the microbiology of venous leg ulcers: a pilot study. J Wound Care 2009;18:164–7.

33. Borgquist O, Gustafsson L, Ingemansson R, et al. Micro- and macromechanical effects on the wound bed of negative pressure wound therapy using gauze and foam. Ann Plast Surg 2010;64:789–93.

34. Weed T, Ratliff C, Drake DB. Quantifying bacterial bioburden during negative pressure wound therapy: does the VAC enhance bacterial clearance? Ann Plast Surg 2004;52:276–9.

35. Mueller SW, Krebsbach LE. Impact of antimicrobial-impregnated gauze dressing on surgical site infections including methicillin-resistant *Staphylococcus aureus* infections. Am J Infect Control 2008;36:651–5.

36. Morykwas MJ, Simpson J, Punger K, et al. Vacuum-assisted closure: state of basic research and physiologic foundation. Plast Reconstr Surg 2006;117:121S–6S.

37. Kamolz LP, Andel H, Haslik W, et al. Use of subatmospheric pressure therapy to prevent burn wound progression in human: first experiences. Burns 2004;30:253–8.

38. Malmsjo M, Ingemansson R, Martin R, et al. Negative-pressure wound therapy using gauze of open-cell polyurethane foam: similar early effects on pressure transduction and tissue contraction in an experimental porcine wound model. Wound Repair Regen 2009;17:200–5.

39. Wysocki AB, Staiano-Coico L, Grinnell F. Wound fluid from chronic leg ulcers contains elevated levels of metalloproteinases MMP-2 and MMP-9. J Invest Dermatol 1993;101:64–8.

40. Tarnuzzer RW, Schultz GS. Biochemical analysis of acute and chronic wound environments. Wound Repair Regen 1996;4:321–5.

41. Mast BA, Schultz GS. Interactions of cytokines, growth factors, and proteases in acute and chronic wounds. Wound Repair Regen 1996;4:411–20.
42. Green AK, Puder M, Roy R, et al. Microdeformational wound therapy: effects on angiogenensis and matrix metalloproteinases in chronic wounds of 3 debilitated patients. Ann Plast Surg 2006;56:418–22.
43. Stechmiller JK, Kilpadi DV, Childress B, et al. Effect of vacuum-assisted closure therapy on the expression of cytokines and proteases in wound fluid of adults with pressure ulcers. Wound Repair Regen 2006;14:371–4.
44. Shi B, Chen SZ, Zhang P, et al. Effects of vacuum-assisted closure (VAC) on the expressions of MMP-1, 2, 13 in human granulation wound. Zhonghua Zheng Xing Wai Ke Za Zhi 2003;19:279–81.
45. KCI therapy clinical guidelines: a reference source for clinicians. Available at: http://www.kci1.com/cs/Satellite?blobcol=urldata&blobheadername1=Content-type&blobheadername2=Content-disposition&blobheadername3=MDT-Type&blobheadervalue1=application%2Fpdf&blobheadervalue2=inline%3B+filename%3D861%252F344%252F2-B-128g_Clinical%252BGuidelines-WEB.pdf&blobheadervalue3=abinary%3B+charset%3DUTF-8&blobkey=id&blobtable=MungoBlobs&blobwhere=1226697053729&ssbinary=true. Accessed December 23, 2014.
46. Fortelny RH, Hofmann A, Gruber-Blum S, et al. Delayed closure of open abdomen in septic patients is facilitated by combined negative pressure wound therapy and dynamic fascial suture. Surg Endosc 2014;28:735–40.
47. Cheatham MI, Demetriades D, Fabian TC, et al. Prospective study examining clinical outcomes associated with a negative pressure wound therapy system and Barker's vacuum packing technique. World J Surg 2013;37:2018–30.
48. Quyn AJ, Johnston C, Hall D, et al. The open abdomen and temporary abdominal closure systems – historical evolution and systematic review. Colorectal Dis 2012; 14:e429–38.
49. Carlson GL, Patrick H, Amin AI, et al. Management of the open abdomen: a national study of clinical outcome and safety of negative pressure wound therapy. Ann Surg 2013;257:1154–9.
50. Lindstedt S, Hlebowicz J. Blood flow response in small intestinal loops at different depths during negative pressure wound therapy of the open abdomen. Int Wound J 2013;10:411–7.
51. Bertelsen CA, Fabricius R, Kleif J, et al. Outcome of negative-pressure wound therapy for open abdomen treatment after nontraumatic lower gastrointestinal surgery: analysis of factors affecting delayed fascial closure in 101 patients. World J Surg 2014;38:774–81.
52. Stannard JP, Gabriel A, Lehner B. Use of negative pressure wound therapy over clean, closed surgical incisions. Int Wound J 2012;9(Suppl 1):32–9.
53. Karlakki S, Bren M, Giannini S, et al. Negative pressure wound therapy for management of the surgical incision in orthopaedic surgery. Bone Joint Res 2013;2: 276–84.
54. Suzuki T, Minehara A, Matsuura T, et al. Negative-pressure wound therapy over surgically closed wounds in open fractures. J Orthop Surg 2014;22:30–4.
55. Davis K, Bills J, Barker J, et al. Simultaneous irrigation and negative pressure wound therapy enhances wound healing and reduces wound bioburden in a porcine model. Wound Repair Regen 2013;21:869–72.
56. Back DA, Scheuermann-Poley C, Willy C. Recommendations on negative pressure wound therapy with installation and antimicrobial solutions – when, where and how to use: what does the evidence show? Int Wound J 2013;10(Suppl 1): 32–42.

57. Rycerz A, Allen D, Lessing MC. Science supporting negative pressure wound therapy with installation. Int Wound J 2013;10(Suppl 1):20–4.
58. Lessing MC, James RB, Ingran SC. Comparison of the effects of different negative pressure wound therapy modes – continuous, noncontinuous, and with installation – on porcine excisional wounds. Eplasty 2013;13:443–54.
59. Brinkert D, Ali M, Naud M, et al. Negative pressure wound therapy with saline installation: 131 patient case series. Int Wound J 2013;10(Suppl 1):56–60.
60. Andrades P, Figueroa M, Sepulveda S, et al. Tumor recurrence after negative pressure wound therapy: an alert call. Case Rep Clin Med 2014;3:350–2.
61. Lehner B, Fleischmann W, Becker R, et al. First experiences with negative pressure wound therapy and installation in the treatment of infected orthopaedic implants: a clinical observational study. Int Orthop 2011;35:1415–20.
62. Leung BK, LaBarbera LA, Carroll CA, et al. The effects of normal saline installation in conjunction with negative pressure wound therapy on wound healing in a porcine model. Wounds 2010;22:179–87.
63. Lessing MC, Slack PS, Hong KZ, et al. Negative pressure wound therapy with controlled saline installation (NPWTI): dressing properties and granulation response in vivo. Wounds 2011;23:309–19.
64. Ahearn C. Intermittent NPWT and lower negative pressures – exploring the disparity between science and current practice: a review. Ostomy Wound Manage 2009;55:22–8.
65. Malmsjo M, Gustafsson L, Lindstedt S, et al. The effects of variable, intermittent, and continuous negative pressure wound therapy, using foam or gauze, on wound contraction, granulation tissue formation, and ingrowth into the wound filler. Eplasty 2012;12:e5.
66. Dastouri P, Helm DL, Scherer SS, et al. Waveform modulation of negative-pressure wound therapy in the murine model. Plast Reconstr Surg 2011;127:1460–6.
67. Kairinos N, Solomons M, Hudson DA. Negative-pressure wound therapy I: the paradox of negative-pressure wound therapy. Plast Reconstr Surg 2009;123:589–98.
68. Birk-Sorensen H, Malmsjo M, Rome P, et al. Evidence-based recommendations for negative pressure wound therapy: treatment variables (pressure levels, wound filler and contact layer) – Steps towards an international concensus. J Plast Reconstr Aesthet Surg 2011;64:S1–16.
69. Fraccalvieri M, Zingarelli E, Ruka E, et al. Negative pressure wound therapy using gauze and foam: histological, immunohistochemical and ultrasonography morphological analysis of the granulation tissue and scar tissue. Preliminary report of a clinical study. Int Wound J 2011;8:355–64.
70. Jeffery SL. Advanced wound therapies in the management of severe military lower limb trauma: a new perspective. Eplasty 2009;21:e28.
71. Hurd T, Chadwick P, Cote J, et al. Impact of gauze-based NPWT on the patient and nursing experience in the treatment of challenging wounds. Int Wound J 2010;7:448–55.
72. Psoinos CM, Ignotz RA, Lalikos JF, et al. Use of a gauze-based negative pressure wound therapy in a pediatric burn patient. J Pediatr Surg 2009;44:e23–6.
73. Malmsjo M, Lindsedt S, Ingemansson R. Effects of foam or gauze on sternum wound contraction, distension and heart and lung damage during negative pressure wound therapy of porcine sternotomy wounds. Interact Cardiovasc Thorac Surg 2011;12:349–54.
74. Dorafshar AH, Franczyk M, Gottlieb LJ, et al. A prospective randomized trial comparing subatmospheric wound therapy with a sealed gauze dressing and the standard vacuum assisted closure device. Ann Plast Surg 2012;69:79–84.

75. Negosanti L, Aceti A, Bianchi T, et al. Adapting a vacuum assisted closure dressing to challenging wounds: negative pressure treatment for perineal necrotizing fasciitis with rectal prolapse in a newborn affected by acute myeloid leukaemia. Eur J Dermatol 2010;20:501–3.

76. Payne JL, Ambrosio AM. Evaluation of an antimicrobial silver foam dressing for use with V.A.C. therapy: morphological, mechanical, and antimicrobial properties. J Biomed Mater Res B Appl Biomater 2009;89:217–22.

77. Gerry R, Kwei S, Bayer L, et al. Silver-impregnated vacuum assisted closure in the treatment of recalcitrant venous stasis ulcers. Ann Plast Surg 2007;59: 58–62.

78. Gabriel A, Heinrich C, Shores J, et al. Reducing bacterial bioburden in infected wounds with vacuum assisted closure and a new silver dressing – a pilot study. Wounds 2006;18:245–55.

79. Borgquist O, Ingemansson R, Malmsjo M. Individualizing the use of negative pressure wound therapy for optimal wound healing: a focused review of the literature. Ostomy Wound Manage 2011;57:44–54.

80. Osterhoff G, Zwolak P, Kruger C, et al. Risk factors for prolonged treatment and hospital readmission in 280 cases of negative-pressure wound therapy. J Plast Reconstr Aesthet Surg 2014;67:629–33.

81. Fieger AJ, Schwatlo F, Mundel DF, et al. Abdominal vacuum therapy for the open abdomen: a retrospective analysis of 82 consecutive patients. Zentralbl Chir 2011;136:56–60.

82. Rao M, Burke D, Finan PJ, et al. The use of vacuum-assisted closure of abdominal wounds: a word of caution. Colorectal Dis 2007;9:266–8.

83. Waldi K. Pain associated with negative pressure wound therapy. Br J Nurs 2013; 22:S15–21.

84. Buote NJ, Havig ME. The use of vacuum-assisted closure in the management of septic peritonitis in six dogs. J Am Anim Hosp Assoc 2012;48:164–71.

85. Cioffi KM, Schmiedt CW, Cornell KK, et al. Retrospective evaluation of vacuum-assisted peritoneal drainage for the treatment of septic peritonitis in dogs and cats: 8 cases (2003-2010). J Vet Emerg Crit Care 2012;22:601–9.

86. Greenfield CL, Walshaw R. Open peritoneal drainage for treatment of contaminated peritoneal cavity and septic peritonitis in dogs and cats: 24 cases (1980–1986). J Am Vet Med Assoc 1987;191:100–5.

87. Woolfson JM, Dulisch ML. Open abdominal drainage in the treatment of generalized peritonitis in 25 dogs and cats. Vet Surg 1986;15:27–32.

88. Hosgood G, Salisbury SK. Generalized peritonitis in dogs: 50 cases (1975–1986). J Am Vet Med Assoc 1988;193:1448–50.

89. Winkler KP, Greenfield CL. Potential prognostic indicators in diffuse peritonitis treated with open peritoneal drainage in the canine patient. Vet Emerg Crit Care 2000;10:259–65.

90. Mueller MG, Ludwig LL, Barton LJ. Use of closed-suction drains to treat generalized peritonitis in dogs and cats: 40 cases (1997-1999). J Am Vet Med Assoc 2001;219:789–94.

91. Wilkes RP, Kilpad DV, Zhao Y, et al. Closed incision management with negative pressure wound therapy (CIM): biomechanics. Surg Innov 2012;19:67–75.

92. Glaser DA, Farnsworth CL, Varley ES, et al. Negative pressure therapy for closed spin incisions: a pilot study. Wounds 2012;24:308–16.

93. Meeker J, Weinhold P, Dahners L. Negative pressure therapy on primarily closed wounds improves wound healing parameters in 3 days in a porcine model. J Orthop Trauma 2011;25:756–61.

94. Hurd T, Trueman P, Rossington A. Use of a portable, single-use negative pressure wound therapy device in home care patients with low to moderately exuding wounds: a case series. Ostomy Wound Manage 2014;60:30–6.

95. Van den Bulck R, Sieberts Y, Zimmer R, et al. Initial clinical experiences with a new, portable, single-use negative pressure wound therapy device. Int Wound J 2013;10:145–51.

96. Hudson DA, Adams KG, Van Huyssteen A, et al. Simplified negative pressure wound therapy: clinical evaluation of an ultraportable, no-canister system. Int Wound J 2013. http://dx.doi.org/10.1111/iwj.12080.

Antimicrobial Considerations in the Perioperative Patient

Dawn Merton Boothe, DVM, PhD[a], Harry W. Boothe Jr, DVM, MS[b],*

KEYWORDS

- Antimicrobial prophylaxis • Surgical site infection • Antiseptics • Disinfectants

KEY POINTS

- Antimicrobial use likely can be de-escalated in the surgical patient.
- Systemic antimicrobial prophylaxis is indicated in the perioperative period only in limited circumstances.
- Antimicrobial dosing regimens should be based on pharmacokinetic/pharmacodynamic indices specific for time-dependent or concentration-dependent drugs.
- The more at risk the patient is to develop antimicrobial resistance, the more important the initial dose and interval of the antimicrobial drug dosing regimen.

Among the most important perioperative considerations for the surgical patient is antimicrobial therapy. The Center for Disease Control Healthcare-Associated Infections (http://www.cdc.gov/hai/) has defined a surgical site infection (SSI) to be one that occurs after surgery in the part of the body where the surgery took place. Potential locations for SSI include superficial or deep incisional and organ or space and may include implanted materials.[1] In human medicine, incidence of SSI varies with the surgical procedure and method of data collection, but it may be as high as 20%.[2] The hospital cost of a patient with an SSI is twice that for one without.[3] The incidence of SSI in dogs and cats is largely unknown. Retrospectively, 3% of dog owners (n = 846) indicated a postoperative SSI (within 30 days) in one study,[4] while another study cites 0.8% to 18% of surgical procedures to be complicated by SSI.[5] Risk factors for SSI have been delineated in humans and include both patient factors (eg, age, nutrition, microbial colonization, and foreign materials at the surgical site, length of preoperative stay) and operative factors (eg, duration of scrub and operation, patient preparation, antimicrobial prophylaxis, environmental considerations).[1] Risk factors in

The Authors have nothing to disclose.
[a] Clinical Pharmacology Laboratory, Department of Anatomy, Physiology and Pharmacology, College of Veterinary Medicine, Auburn University, 1130 Wire Road, Auburn, AL 36849, USA;
[b] Department of Clinical Sciences, College of Veterinary Medicine, Auburn University, 1220 Wire Road, Auburn, AL 36849, USA
* Corresponding author.
E-mail address: boothhw@auburn.edu

Vet Clin Small Anim 45 (2015) 585–608
http://dx.doi.org/10.1016/j.cvsm.2015.01.006
0195-5616/15/$ – see front matter © 2015 Elsevier Inc. All rights reserved.
vetsmall.theclinics.com

veterinary patients should be anticipated to be similar. Singh and colleagues[5] identified significant factors to be implant placement, intraoperative hypotension, and surgical classification (clean vs dirty). Nazarali and colleagues[6] found anesthesia time to be a risk factor for SSI. The risk of an SSI is increased if greater than 10^5 colony forming units (CFU) are present per gram of tissue, although the number may be as low as 10^2 for staphylococci.[1] Immune suppression is a likely risk factor in veterinary medicine, because an infection rate of 26% was reported within 8 days (before discharge) after renal transplantation (ie, before discharge) in cats.[7]

Presumably, the incidence of SSI might be decreased by implementation of timely, appropriate antimicrobial therapy. Determinations of appropriateness include, among other considerations, the microbial target and a properly designed dosing regimen to minimize the likelihood of a residual, resistant, infecting inoculum is left at the site. The greater the risk that the patient is unable to overcome a residual population due to systemic or local immune-incompetence or other factors, the more diligent the surgeon should be in the implementation of antimicrobial therapy. This article focuses on several key approaches to the rational, judicious use of antibacterials in the perioperative surgical patient using a 3-D approach: de-escalation of antimicrobial use, design of a dosing regimen to kill the entire infecting incoculum, and decontamination of the patient, surgeon, and environment.

DE-ESCALATING ANTIMICROBIAL USE

Inappropriate perioperative antimicrobial use increases the incidence of complications. Examples of inappropriate perioperative antimicrobial use include use of antimicrobials for clean surgical procedures, initiation of prophylactic antimicrobials postoperatively, and continuation of antimicrobial administration for longer than 24 hours. Antimicrobial use facilitates emerging resistance not only through selection pressure (survival of the fittest) but also through phenotypic changes that occur in the infecting microbial population.[8] Recent studies in dogs have demonstrated that systemic antimicrobial therapy, whether oral (amoxicillin, enrofloxacin)[9] or injectable (cefovecin[9]), is associated with emergent resistance to the treatment drug in fecal *Escherichia coli* or *Enterococcus* spp. Such findings further support de-escalation of antimicrobial use as an approach to decrease the risk of resistance in the surgical patient. Thus, the first and perhaps single most important decision to be made regarding antimicrobial therapy in the surgical patient is whether systemic antimicrobial prophylaxis is indicated.

Antimicrobial Prophylaxis

Surgical antimicrobial prophylaxis involves a brief course of an antimicrobial drug initiated just before an operation begins, in the absence of infection.[1] Guidelines for prophylaxis have been promulgated in humans,[1,10] with the more recent guidelines providing criteria for strength of evidence.[10] The goal of antimicrobial prophylaxis in the surgical patient is not sterilization of tissues, but rather the reduction of microbial burden and the risk of intraoperative contamination such that normal host defenses can prevent infection. Prophylaxis is distinguished from treatment in that the latter is implemented in response to bacterial contamination (eg, an open fracture, contamination of abdominal contents with intestinal fluid).

Antimicrobial prophylaxis is not a substitute for good surgical practices. If implemented in anticipation of an invasive procedure (ie, surgery), the following factors should serve as a basis for implementing antimicrobial prophylaxis: surgery type, the pathogens most likely to be encountered during the procedure, and drug safety. The chosen drug should have demonstrated efficacy for prophylaxis. The dosing regimen should be designed to achieve the recommended pharmacodynamic/pharmacokinetic index (PKPDI) for the drug such that adequate bactericidal drug concentrations are achieved and maintained at the site of invasion before potential contamination and until shortly after completion of surgery. As such, if a time-dependent antimicrobial drug is used, it should either have a long elimination half-life or be re-dosed during lengthy procedures. In addition, the duration of therapy should be as short as possible.[11–13]

Prophylactic antimicrobial therapy is not warranted for most clean procedures for which bacterial contamination is expected to be minor. An exception might be surgeries for which surgical implants are used or if consequences of infection would be catastrophic (eg, total joint replacement). Clean-contaminated surgeries (eg, gastrointestinal, genitourinary, respiratory), or procedures in which a break in sterile technique occurred without significant intraoperative spillage, may benefit from prophylactic antimicrobial therapy.

Antimicrobial prophylaxis is generally warranted when surgery is classified as contaminated (eg, presence of acute, nonpurulent inflammation or gross contamination from a hollow viscus). Extensive tissue damage or accumulation of blood within wounds facilitates bacterial colonization, generally warranting prophylactic antimicrobial drug administration. Such wounds might benefit from irrigation with antiseptics. Chlorhexidine (0.05%) is an effective antiseptic for infected wounds. Use of antimicrobials (systemically, topically, or both) is generally indicated before surgery to treat an infected or dirty wound. Such use is more appropriately termed therapeutic antimicrobial therapy.

Identifying the antimicrobial target and source of antimicrobial prophylaxis can be problematic. Endogenous bacterial sources (eg, skin, mucosa) probably play a greater role in postoperative infections than exogenous sources. Hematogenous spread of bacteria from overt or occult septic foci or dental manipulation is a concern. Ideally, such sources should be either eliminated before surgery by appropriate therapeutic antimicrobial agents or avoided by not combining dental manipulations with surgery of body cavities or orthopedic procedures.

The most frequently encountered pathogenic bacterial contaminants of surgical wounds to be targeted by prophylactic antimicrobials are *Staphylococcus* spp and *E coli*. In humans, the most frequent pathogens and their percentages reported were *Staphylococcus* spp (34%), *Enterococcus* spp (12%), *E coli* and *Pseudomonas aeruginosa* (8% each), and *Enterobacter* spp (7%).[1] *Staphylococcus pseudintermedius* was the most commonly identified diagnosed organism in veterinary patients.[5] Thirteen percent of dogs undergoing tibial plateau leveling osteotomy developed a SSI, with *S pseudintermedius* found in 88% of the positive cultures, and 40% being methicillin resistant.[6] *Enterococcus* spp, which are resistant to cephalosporins, and *E coli* made up smaller percentages. By site, the most common skin bacteria are *Staphylococcus* spp, although many other organisms may be present as transient, topical flora. The oropharynx has a mixed population of gram-positive (especially *Staphylococcus* spp, *Streptococcus* spp, and *Actinomyces pyogenes*), gram-negative (*Proteus* spp, *Pasteurella* spp, *Pseudomonas* spp, and *E coli*), and anaerobic organisms. The stomach and proximal small intestine normally have very few organisms, whereas the distal ileum and large intestine have large numbers of gram-negative (especially *E coli*, *Klebsiella* spp, *Pseudomonas* spp, and *Salmonella* spp) and anaerobic organisms. Potential pathogens encountered in the genitourinary tract include both gram-positive and gram-negative organisms (especially *Staphylococcus* and *Streptococcus* spp, *E coli*, and *Proteus* and *Pseudomonas* spp). Pathogens of the respiratory tract (especially lower respiratory tract) include both gram-positive (*Staphylococcus* spp, *Streptococcus* spp, and *A pyogenes*) and gram-negative organisms (*Pseudomonas* spp, *E coli*, and *Klebsiella*, *Pasteurella*, and *Enterobacter* spp).

The selected antimicrobial should be bactericidal for the pathogens that are most likely to be encountered. First-generation cephalosporins (eg, cefazolin) are generally as effective as and less expensive than second-generation and third-generation cephalosporins. Surgery of the lower gastrointestinal tract may require a more elaborate schedule of prophylactic antimicrobial administration, partly because of the presence of anaerobic organisms. A second-generation cephalosporin (eg, cefoxitin) or an aminoglycoside/anaerobic combination (eg, amikacin or gentamicin with clindamycin, amoxicillin, or metronidazole) should be administered systemically. The use of oral antimicrobials for prophylaxis may not be prudent, in part, because peak concentrations are likely to be lower than with intravenous (IV) administration, even with 100% bioavailability.

The ability to predict antimicrobial efficacy against commonly cited surgical pathogens increasingly is limited. Both *E coli* and *S pseudintermedius* or *S aureus* exhibit increasingly higher minimum inhibitory concentrations (MIC). Thungrat and colleagues[14] demonstrated that canine and feline nonuropathogenic *E coli* were generally more resistant to most antimicrobials tested compared with uropathogic *E coli*. For individual antimicrobials, essentially 100% of isolates were resistant to the first tier antimicrobial cephalothin (the model drug for cephalexin), whereas only 9% expressed resistance to cefazolin. The percentage of isolates resistant to the third-generation drug, cefovecin, was not reported, although 13% of isolates were resistant to cefpodoxime, also a third-generation cephalosporin. Approximately 40% of isolates were resistant to amoxicillin-clavulanic acid and 50% of isolates were resistant to amoxicillin (modeled by ampicillin), suggesting empirical use of amoxicillin-clavulanic acid offers no advantage over amoxicillin alone when treating *E coli*. The likelihood that a common pathogen has developed resistance to these first tier antimicrobials (cephalexin, amoxicillin, and amoxicillin-clavulanic acid) is increased in a patient previously exposed to antimicrobial drugs. Another clinically important finding by Thungrat and colleagues[14] is that many "susceptible" isolates are characterized by MIC that approach the threshold of susceptibility, indicating some level of resistance has emerged; this indicates that antimicrobial doses routinely should be high, and for time-dependent drugs, intervals may need to be shortened.

For *Staphylococcus* spp, although the information is not as robust, evidence indicates that methicillin resistance is rapidly emerging in both *S pseudintermedius* and *S aureus*, as was reviewed by Weese and van Duijkeren.[15] Using antibiograms at Auburn University, during 2003 to 2005, the percentages of *S pseudintermedius* and *S aureus* resistant to cephalexin (modeled by cephalothin) and amoxicillin-clavulanic acid were 4% and 40%, respectively. Between 2007 and 2010, those numbers had increased to 22% and 53%, respectively, because of methicillin resistance. By 2012, methicillin resistance of *S pseudintermedius* had increased to 43%. Interestingly, methicillin resistance of *S aureus* had decreased to 23%, although the sample size was small.

Because the primary goal of antimicrobial prophylaxis is to achieve bactericidal concentrations at the surgical site by the time of wound contamination, factors influencing the design of dosing regimens for perioperative antimicrobials should be considered. Such factors include timing and route of administration, and drug absorption, distribution, and elimination. Hawn and colleagues[16] demonstrated that the incidence of SSI was higher in human patients that received antimicrobials after 60 minutes, compared with 60 minutes or less, before surgical incision. A similar tendency was found in dogs undergoing an orthopedic procedure.[6] IV antimicrobial administration is recommended to achieve the highest concentrations of drug most rapidly, eliminating concerns about drug absorption. For most antimicrobials, tissue distribution is relatively rapid, being complete in most tissues within 30 to 60 minutes after IV administration. The concentration of antimicrobial achieved in the tissue correlates with the concentration of free drug in the serum. Highly protein-bound antimicrobials (eg, cefovecin) achieve lower tissue compared with plasma drug concentrations than do weakly bound antimicrobials (eg, cefazolin, gentamicin, ampicillin). Time to peak tissue antimicrobial concentrations also may be delayed by high serum protein binding. For example, peak serum and transudate (interstitial fluid) cefovecin concentrations occurred at 3 hours and 2.5 days, respectively. Based on pharmacodynamic antimicrobial activity (reduction in S pseudintermedius CFU), cefovecin effects are not evident in transudate until 4 hours, with peak activity occurring at 2.5 days.[17] The antimicrobial may become rebound, and thus inactivated, to inflammatory proteins in tissue, decreasing efficacy while prolonging its presence. Antimicrobial activity of cefovecin at day 10 was still equal to peak activity and at day 18, approximated 50% of peak activity, precluding a short duration of effect.[17] Accordingly, cefovecin seemingly does not meet the criteria for surgical prophylaxis.

Other factors (eg, lipid solubility, pH, local environment) may also influence tissue penetration or accumulation of antimicrobials. Elimination of most antimicrobials used prophylactically is renal. The rate of elimination determines elimination half-life, which in turn determines the dosing interval of time-dependent drugs. More rapidly eliminated drugs require more frequent administration. Cefazolin, for example, has an elimination half-life of approximately 1 hour in dogs and, accordingly, should be administered at less than 2-hour intervals during the surgical procedure to maintain adequate tissue and serum levels.

Recommended prophylactic dosing regimens for a variety of surgical interventions have been delineated in humans.[10] For example, a protocol for cefazolin that may be appropriate for a patient not previously exposed to antimicrobials is an initial IV dose given 10 to 30 minutes before incision (ie, at anesthetic induction) and a second dose given at the completion of the procedure. If the surgical procedure lasts longer than 2 hours, an additional intraoperative dose should be given approximately 90 minutes after the initial dose. The risk of bacterial contamination continues until a fibrin seal develops across wound edges (approximately 3–5 hours postoperatively). After that time period, continuation of antimicrobial administration has no scientific rationale. However, with documented infection, therapeutic antimicrobial therapy is initiated.

Evidence for the role of prophylactic antimicrobial therapy in preventing SSI can be found in both veterinary and human medicine. Although surgical prophylaxis has been integrated into the perioperative surgical plans for veterinary patients, relatively little information supports its use. In one controlled study of dogs (n = 329) and cats (n = 544) undergoing clean and clean-contaminated surgical procedures, the postoperative infection rate did not differ in placebo (9.4%) compared with the cephalexin-pretreated group (8.9%).[18] In another study investigating the impact of tympanic cavity flushing in dogs undergoing total ear canal ablation, isolates were characterized by a relatively higher incidence of antimicrobial resistance to cefazolin (20%[19]), suggesting that cefazolin may not be a rational choice in all presurgical candidates. Eugster and colleagues[13] prospectively examined risk factors for SSI in dogs and cats. Animals were treated with cephalexin IV (20 mg/kg) at induction and then every 3 hours until surgery ended. Infected animals (contaminated or dirty procedures) were treated with various antimicrobials. Antimicrobial use influenced the risk of SSI in this study. Notably, of the 735 animals studied, 92% (clean) to 95% (contaminated) of animals received perioperative prophylactic therapy. Because the number of animals not receiving antimicrobials was so small, the statistical analysis was limited. However, preoperative and postoperative administration of antimicrobials were "associated with an increased frequency of SSI," with antimicrobial prophylaxis providing "some protection against surgical wound infections." Based on their findings, the authors indicate that preoperative and intraoperative antimicrobial prophylaxis represented an important protective factor.

Topical and Local Antimicrobial Prophylaxis

Among the approaches to de-escalate antimicrobial prophylaxis is topical or local antimicrobial administration at the incision site. This approach has been reviewed in human medicine.[20,21] Among the advantages of local antibiotic administration include high, and potentially sustained, concentrations at the site of infection, the potential for limited risk of systemic toxicity, and a reduced risk of antimicrobial resistance.[20] Among the biggest disadvantages is the lack of guidelines and evidence of efficacy. Other disadvantages include the potential for impaired surgical wound healing, and local hypersensitivity. In general, as with systemic prophylaxis, local therapy should be considered particularly when benefits outweigh risks (eg, procedures with a high rate of infection, or when the sequelae of infection are disastrous).

In humans, the most commonly used local antimicrobials are cephalosporins, aminoglycosides, glycopeptides, chloramphenicol, and bacitracin. Methods of delivery include intraoperative washes, injections, locally applied lotions, solutions, powders, gels, creams, or ointments, and antimicrobial implanted beads or implants.[21] Variability in drug, method delivery, and the unique pharmacokinetic and pharmacodynamics characteristics of the drugs used limits the ability to compare studies and come to consensus regarding topical or local prophylaxis. Note that failure of a study to demonstrate a significant difference between 2 or more treatment groups cannot be interpreted as evidence of lack of efficacy; rather, for many of these studies, insufficient sample size resulted in failure to demonstrate a significant difference in the face of outcome variability.[10]

For orthopedic procedures, IV administration is recommended. Although animal studies indicate that antimicrobial irrigation fluids used during surgery reduced SSI, more recent studies involving clinical trials indicate no potential benefit of such solutions used to remove staphylococci from stainless steel screws.[20,21]

Among the methods of local antimicrobial delivery studied for orthopedic procedures is local placement of antimicrobial-impregnated cement or beads for in bone, synovial structures, and other soft tissues. Indications include refractory infections, particularly osteomyelitis, and prophylaxis after surgery of contaminated wounds. Although many animal and clinical studies have been implemented, conclusions of clinical trials are limited by small sample size.[20,21]

Antimicrobial-impregnated beads have been studied in veterinary medicine for treatment or prevention of osteomyelitis.[22–25] Two forms of beads have been used: polymethyl methacrylate (PMMA) and, more recently, calcium-based (eg, sulfate, plaster of Paris) beads. Both are prepared by mixing drug in the powder form and then sterilizing the bead using a non–heat-based method. The major difference between the 2 beads is that the PMMA beads are not biodegradable, thus requiring a second surgery for removal. Furthermore, their preparation results in an exothermic process that requires heat-stable antimicrobials and may cause host tissue damage or decreased host phagocytic function. Calcium-based beads are biodegradable and not exothermic. An additional advantage of calcium sulfate is osteoconduction, which potentially facilitates bone healing. Several commercially available PMMA cements are available; in addition, compounding pharmacies are beginning to offer antimicrobial-impregnated beads.

Regardless of the matrix type, in vitro studies demonstrate that the release or elution of antimicrobial from beads is bimodal, characterized by an initial rapid release (lasting 12–48 hours) followed by a slower release that may extend to weeks or months. Generally, therapeutic concentrations can be anticipated for up to 10 days.[21-23] For PMMA, elution rates (based on in vitro studies) vary with antimicrobial concentration in the bead, pore, and bead size, and permeability of the cement (which, in turn, can be affected by the amount and type of antimicrobial). The form (eg, liquid vs powder) of the antimicrobial also influences elution rates. Host factors influencing elution rates include surface area available for bead exposure, blood flow, and fluid content. Atilla[22] and others[23] have demonstrated that the combination of drugs in beads increases the elution rate and may not be recommended. In general, concentrations in the first stage of elution surrounding the area can be anticipated to exceed the MIC_{90} of most susceptible organisms by more than a hundred-fold, increasing the likelihood of a quick kill. Concentrations during the second phase of elution will be much lower but may still surpass the MIC_{90} of infecting microbes. Atilla[22] also demonstrated that the elution rate may increase even if drugs are not mixed in the same bead but are in different beads.

A commonality of in vitro drug elution studies is their questionable applicability to drug elution in the patient. Studies ideally are based on concentrations measured in vivo using ultrafiltration probes that collect interstitial fluid. For example, in his review, Sayegh[25] reported that encapsulation of the beads during healing results in therapeutic concentrations being achieved up to 2 to 3 mm surrounding the beads.

Antibiotic-impregnated bead use has been studied in dogs. The use of tobramycin antimicrobial-impregnated calcium sulfate beads in a series of 6 dogs has been recently reported.[24] The beads are commercially available, being approved for use as a bone filler. Sites included forelimb and hind limbs, and infecting organisms included S intermedius, S aureus, and P aeruginosa. Beads generally lost their radio-opacity by 4 weeks and were no longer visible radiographically by 6 to 8 weeks. Clinical signs associated with infection resolved in all but one dog.

Antibiotic-impregnated cement is common practice in human surgeries involving joint arthroplasty.[20] It has been demonstrated to prevent infection with many organisms in rat models. Furthermore, as reviewed by McHugh and colleagues,[20] a meta-analysis found that SSIs in humans were decreased with the use of antibiotic-impregnated cement. Several studies in animal models and humans have failed to demonstrate efficacy of antibiotic-impregnated beads compared with IV antimicrobial administration.[20] However, gentamicin-impregnated beads coupled with IV therapy substantively decreased the rate of SSI in humans (from 12% to 3.7%) compared with patients receiving the drug in beads alone.[20]

Although current human guidelines indicate that evidence exists to support the use of cement in arthroplasties, insufficient evidence exists to support routine use of antimicrobial-impregnated beads in open fracture surgery.[20,21] The potential risks for adversities associated with antimicrobial-impregnated beads or cement need to be further addressed. For example, host response to the cement may facilitate infection by S aureus. In a series of human patients (n = 20), cultures of gentamicin-loaded beads removed 2 weeks after implantation from prosthesis-related infections revealed 90% to be infected. Of the 28 isolates, nearly 70% were gentamicin-resistant.[26] Interestingly, 12 of the 18 infected patients were considered infection free before removal of the infected beads. Most common isolates were P aeruginosa and S aureus. In contrast, the prosthetic devices in the area of the beads tended to not be infected. An additional risk is potential systemic toxicity from the antimicrobial. This risk is greatest with aminoglycosides and has been reported in human medicine (as reviewed by Huiras and colleagues).[21]

Other antimicrobial-impregnated matrices are under investigation, with a focus on those that slowly release the antimicrobial or are biodegradable. One case report describes the successful use of a commercially available gentamicin-impregnated collagen sponge (CollaRx) in the treatment of septic arthritis associated with methicillin-resistant S aureus in a dog.[27] Collagen has the advantage of being biodegradable with release of antimicrobials generally ending 48 to 72 hours after administration.[21]

For abdominal surgery, studies comparing abdominal infusion versus IV administration of intraoperative antimicrobials are largely limited by small sample size. Studies involving gentamicin-infused collagen sponges actually demonstrated an increased risk of SSI, potentially because of the mechanical effects of the sponge. It was noted that a single bolus treatment of gentamicin might be insufficient for prevention of infection by Staphlococcus spp, but not gram-negative bacilli. For abdominal infections, local infusion appears to have demonstrated efficacy only in morbidly obese patients.[10]

For cardiothoracic surgery, systemic prophylaxis is recommended. However, topical vancomycin might be more prudent than β-lactams. As reviewed by Bratzler and colleagues,[10] one study demonstrated that antimicrobial-impregnated collagen reduced the incidence of sternal SSI. Another study found that intracavitary instillation of penicillin G, bacitracin, and gentamicin decreased the incidence of empyema.[10]

For dermatologic procedures, systemic prophylaxis is reserved for high-risk patients.[10] Chloramphenicol ophthalmic ointment is a common preparation used for plastic surgical procedures. For burn patients, systemic antimicrobials seemed to reduce overall mortality in one study, but statistical reduction in SSI was limited. Topical antimicrobials also were not demonstrated to be effective.[10] Note that systemic absorption of topically applied antimicrobials may result in toxicity. This risk is of particular concern with aminoglycosides. Drug-induced nephrotoxicity has been demonstrated in a cat with a subcutaneous infection that was topically treated with gentamicin.[28]

With ocular surgery, multiple blood-tissue barriers exist (ocular, retinal, aqueous) to ocular penetration following systemic antimicrobial therapy, particularly for water-soluble drugs (eg, aminoglycosides, βlactams, and glycopeptides). Accordingly, preoperative conjunctival irrigation with 5% povidone-iodine solution is recommended for prophylaxis for intraocular surgery.[10] To achieve intraocular concentrations, intracameral or subconjunctival administration may be indicated for prevention of SSI.

DESIGNING THE DOSING REGIMEN

Once the decision is made to use systemic antimicrobials, whether prophylactic or therapeutic, the next challenge is designing the dosing regimen such that all infecting colonies are removed. Traditionally, dosing regimens have been chosen to maximize efficacy with little consideration for avoiding resistance. However, given the profound impact that antimicrobial resistance has on therapeutic success with antimicrobials,[29] designing the regimen such that emergent resistance is minimized should also be an objective. Given the profound challenges associated with antimicrobial resistance, a review of the current approaches to systemic antimicrobial therapy is appropriate. Several excellent reviews have addressed the importance of the relationship between plasma drug concentrations, MIC, and antimicrobial efficacy. Among them, Mouton and colleagues[30] and Martinez and colleagues[31] address the importance of achieving targeted PKPDIs for either time-dependent or concentration-dependent antimicrobials using a "hitting hard and fast and getting out quick" approach.

Determining and Achieving Target Pharmacokinetic/Pharmacodynamic Indices

Efficacy of antimicrobials can be enhanced if targeted PKPDI are achieved at the site of infection. These indices describe the relationship between the time course of a drug, measured, for example, by the area under the curve (AUC) or maximum drug concentration (C_{max}) during a 24-hour dosing period, the potency of the antimicrobial against the target microbe (measured, for example, by drug MIC), and the drug efficacy. Traditionally, antimicrobials are referred to as either concentration-dependent or time-dependent. Efficacy of concentration-dependent antimicrobials is enhanced by the magnitude of exposure measured as either AUC/MIC (eg, fluoroquinolones) or C_{max}/MIC (eg., aminoglycosides or fluoroquinolones). Efficacy of time-dependent drugs (eg, cell wall inhibitors, sulfonamides with or without a potentiator, and most single subunit ribosomal inhibitors) depends on duration of exposure and is generally determined by the time that antimicrobials are higher than the isolate MIC (T > MIC). However, efficacy of some time-dependent antimicrobials is based on AUC/MIC; examples include those drugs that exhibit a long postantibiotic effect (eg, most macrolides, clindamycin, and the glycopeptides such as vancomycin). All 3 indices (C_{max}/MIC, T > MIC, and AUC/MIC) depend on antimicrobial drugs at the site of infection being above the MIC. As such, dose is important for all drugs. For concentration-dependent antimicrobials, increasing the dose is the best way to increase C_{max}/MIC or AUC/MIC. Ideally, a C_{max}/MIC $\geq$10 or more is desirable for concentration-dependent drugs. For time-dependent antimicrobials, T > MIC and AUC/MIC are also influenced by drug-elimination half-life. For T > MIC, each doubling of the dose adds an elimination half-life to the duration that drug concentrations are above the MIC. In general, the lower the tier of the antimicrobial, the longer the duration that antimicrobial concentrations should be above the MIC (the longer T > MIC).

The guidelines for targeted PKPDIs for concentration-dependent or time-dependent drugs focus on improving efficacy. However, to avoid emerging resistance, greater magnitudes (higher C_{max}/MIC or longer T > MIC) generally are necessary to minimize the advent of resistance.

Table 1 demonstrates how MIC might be used as a basis for both selecting a drug and designing dosing regimens. When using amoxicillin-clavulanic acid and cephalexin (modeled by cephalothin), the data demonstrate that the T > MIC for amoxicillin-clavulanic acid would only be 3 hours, but for cephalexin, it would be 9 to 15 hours, despite the fact that both isolates are considered "S." The data further demonstrate that ciprofloxacin at 40 mg/kg achieves a C_{max}/MIC ratio of less than 6.6. However, if enrofloxacin is administered at 20 mg/kg, the ratio is 8 (and 14 if ciprofloxacin bioactivity is added to enrofloxacin). As such, enrofloxacin would be the better drug, even though both antimicrobials are designated as "S."

Attention to dosing regimens must be increased if designed to minimize the risk of emerging resistance. Several important factors impact the likelihood of resistance. The size of an infecting inoculum is important. The population in an infection associated with clinical signs often exceeds 10^8 CFU, yet susceptibility testing is generally based on 10^5 CFU. The larger the inoculum size, the more likely that antimicrobial therapy will fail, for at least 3 reasons. First, more isolates mean more microbial targets are present and thus more drug molecules must be present to effectively inhibit the entire infecting population. Second, more CFU means more destructive enzymes (eg, β-lactamases) are likely to be present. Third, the larger the inoculum, the greater the likelihood that spontaneous mutation will result in a CFU that is resistant to the chosen antimicrobial.

An infecting resident population is characterized by a range of MIC. Statistically, the MIC yielded from susceptibility testing is likely to represent be the median or MIC_{50}. As

Table 1
Pharmacokinetic-pharmacodynamics indices in the dog for drugs to which S aureus has demonstrated susceptibility based on minimum inhibitory concentrations as determined by susceptibility testing

	Pharmaco-dynamics		Drug Information				Pharmacokinetics				PKPDI Targets		
Drug	MIC (µg/mL)	Int	Cidal vs Static	Concentration vs Time	Tier 1-4	Dose (mg/kg)	C_{max} (µg/mL)	$t_{1/2}$ (h)	C_{max}/MIC	C_{max}/MIC (≥10)	$T > MIC$ Half-lives	$T > MIC$ (h)
Amikacin[a]	≤2[b]	S	Cidal	Conc	3-4	22 (IV)	65	1-2	≥32	≥32		
Amoxi-clav	≤0.5	I	Cidal	Time	1	12.5	4.5	1.25	≥9	3	3	3
Ampicillin	≥0.5	R	Cidal	Time	1	30	10					
Cephalothin[c]	2	S	Cidal	Time	1	20	20	2-3	10		3	6-9
Ceftazidime[a]	4	S	Cidal	Time	2-3	20	49	1	12		3	3
Cefpodoxime	0.25	S	Cidal	Time	2	5	8.2	5.5	22		4	22
Ceftiofur[a]	1	S	Cidal	Time	2	2.2	8.9	6	9		3	18
Chloramphenicol	1	S	Static	Time	2	20	23	2.5	23		4	10
Ciprofloxacin	1	I	Static	Conc	3	20	2.8	5.3	2.8	2.8		
Clindamycin	0.5	S	Static	Time	1-2	11	5	5	10		3	15
Enrofloxacin	≤0.5	S	Cidal	Conc	2	20	4.2 (7)[d]	4.1	≥8 (≥14[d])	≥8 (≥14[d])		
Azithromycin	0.5	S	Static	Time	2	10	4.9	35	10	NR	8	>24[e]
Gentamicin[a]	0.5	S	Cidal	Conc	2-3	10 (IV)	28	1	56	56		
Meropenem[a]	0.5	S	Cidal	Time	4	20 (IV)	60	0.75	120	240	7	5
Oxacillin		S	Static									

Penicillin	≥0.25	R	Cidal	Time	20,000 IU (IV)	30						
Rifampin	≤1	S	Cidal	Time	3	10	40	9	8	40	5	>24
Tetracycline	4	S	Static	Time	1	20	9	10	2		1	10
Trimethoprim-sulfamethoxazole	1	S	Cidal	Time	1–2	55[f]	67	13	67		6	>24
Vancomycin[a]	1	S	Cidal	Time	4	15 (IV)	40	5	40		5	24

[a] Injectable only.

[b] Less than or equal to indicates the lowest concentration that was tested. The MIC is at or below this concentration. Accordingly, this concentration is used for determination of PKPDI.

[c] Model for cephalexin.

[d] If ciprofloxacin bioactivity is added: 7.0.

[e] Because PKPDI are based on 24 h, T > MIC that exceed 24 h are reported as greater than 24 h. The maximum dosing interval for those patients ideally will be 24 h.

[f] This S aureus isolate was cultured from an intraoperative tissue sample collected 3 weeks postoperatively in a dog with osteomyelitis associated with an external fixation device. Pharmacodynamic information is based on the MIC determined for that isolate. Pharmacokinetic information is based on either the maximum plasma drug concentration (C_{max}) at the dose delineated in the table or the elimination half-life, both of which are specific for the target species (ie, dog). For concentration-dependent drugs, the target PKPDI is a C_{max}:MIC that exceeds 10. For time-dependent drugs, the T > MIC, and thus dosing interval, also depends on the antimicrobial half-life. For each doubling of C_{max}:MIC, the T > MIC is one half-life. Thus, the duration that T > MIC (hour) is the number of half-lives times the half-life of that antimicrobial in the target species. The duration of the dosing interval is based on the T > MIC. For drugs with a longer postantibiotic effect (eg, vancomycin, tetracyclines), the T > MIC might be as little as 25% of the dosing interval, whereas for drugs with minimal PAE (eg, lower-tier β-lactams), the duration may need to be 100% of the dosing interval. Note that patient, disease, or drug factors may necessitate doses that are higher than that necessary to simply achieve targeted plasma PKPDI to minimize the advent of resistance (see text).

such, the MIC on the culture report may not represent the entire infecting inoculum. The mutant prevention concentration (MPC) is the highest MIC, or the MIC_{100} of the infecting population. It is this MIC that should be the target if the entire infecting inoculum is to be inhibited. The mutant selection window is described by the MIC reported on the susceptibility report (lower threshold) and the highest MIC in the infecting population (higher threshold). If dosing regimens result in antimicrobial concentrations that are less than the MPC, those CFU that are not inhibited are resistant to the antimicrobial at the dose used. For an immune-competent patient, this residual, resistant inoculum is likely to be eradicated. However, the more immune-incompetent the patient is (or the greater "at risk" the patient is for resistance), the more likely this residual, resistant inoculum will multiply and emerge to become a resistant infection. Unfortunately, the MPC of antimicrobials cannot be predicted based on MIC. Liu and colleagues[32] demonstrated that the MPC for enrofloxacin approximated 10 times the MIC for *E coli*, but other studies have demonstrated much higher MPC:MIC ratios, particularly for gram-positive isolates.

Martinez and colleagues[31] also emphasize the importance of the first dose of an antimicrobial and the necessity of avoiding suboptimal drug exposure, thus promoting a "hit quick" component to the therapy. A quick, hard hit will decrease the inoculum size, thus minimizing rather than facilitating emergent resistance. Both Mouton and colleagues[30] and Martinez and colleagues[31] emphasize the importance of short rather than longer durations of therapy to minimize resistance. In general, a dosing regimen that is 4 to 5 days is sufficient for efficacy (assuming proper dosing regimens are used) and appears to minimize amplification of resistance. In contrast, dosing regimens that extend to 10 days will facilitate therapeutic failure due to an emergent resistant population.[30,31] Constant and prolonged antimicrobial exposure may facilitate emergence of a dormant, persistent cell state (see later discussion).[31] Studies have demonstrated that resistant colonies increasingly comprise a greater proportion of the total infecting (residual) population as duration of antimicrobial exposure increases; this proportion increases if suboptimal drug concentrations are achieved at the site. The longer the duration of therapy, the greater the drug exposure must be to suppress emergent resistant populations. These findings support the "get out quick" approach to antimicrobial therapy. Furthermore, combined, these data support the exploration of unconventional dosing regimens that might minimize antimicrobial resistance, such as pulse dosing, dosing with initially higher doses (frontloading), or shortened durations.

Drug Distribution to Site of Infection

Many other factors influence the relationship between plasma drug concentrations and MIC. Among those most relevant to the surgical patient are drug distribution to the site of infection and biofilm. Sinusoidal capillaries, found primarily in the adrenal cortex, pituitary gland, liver, and spleen, present essentially no barrier to drug movement. Fenestrated capillaries such as those located in kidneys and endocrine glands contain pores that facilitate rapid distribution of unbound drug between plasma and interstitium. Muscle, lungs, and adipose tissue contain continuous capillaries and thus may present some level of barrier to drug movement.[33–35] However, other continuous capillaries, such as those found in the brain, eye, cerebrospinal fluid, testes, and prostate, present a major barrier to drug movement due to endothelial cells with tight junctions.[33] Therapeutic antimicrobial failure in humans has been associated with failed drug penetration, including soft tissue infections, osteomyelitis, prostatitis, otitis, endocarditis, ocular infections, periodontitis, and sinusitis. Such failures presumably reflect, in part, failed antimicrobial delivery.[34]

Models for the detection of drugs in tissues should focus on interstitial (extracellular) concentrations.[35,36] Methods that measure concentrations in tissue homogenates (including both intracellular and extracellular fluid) do not accurately represent interstitial concentrations. Detection of drug in fluids is often based on methods that require at least 1 mL or more of fluid. Determination of drug in tissues protected by specialized barriers is difficult, generally requiring anesthesia.[37] However, extracellular fluids can be collected by a variety of methods. Among them, models based on ultrafiltration techniques appear to be most accurate representations of extracellular fluid in the normal animal.[38] Comparison to plasma data must be based on the entire time versus concentration curve (ie, AUC, C_{max}) rather than single-point comparisons, because drug does not distribute immediately into tissues. Care must also be taken to address the impact of protein binding, as can be demonstrated for cefovecin, a drug that is 90% to 99% bound to serum protein. Total serum concentrations are markedly higher than that in extracellular fluid because the latter contains less protein.[17] However, an increase in inflammation may influence distribution into tissues because of increased protein or changes in environmental pH, both of which may increase the proportion of nondiffusible drug in extracellular tissue.

Based on the above caveats with most studies using ultrafiltration or microdialysis techniques, interstitial concentrations of most drugs in most tissues parallel that in plasma, with relative bioavailability based on AUC generally approximating 70% to 100% (**Table 2**). Antimicrobials characterized by larger volumes of distribution for unbound drug (eg, fluoroquinolones) are characterized by relative bioavailability in interstitial fluid of skeletal muscle or subcutaneous interstitial that exceed unity. This finding is also true for enrofloxacin versus cefazolin or metronidazole in canine peritoneal or medullary cavity concentrations (Boothe DM, Boothe HW, 2007, unpublished data). Distribution of β-lactams frequently approaches unity, although site and route make a difference. For example, for amoxicillin, distribution to superficial skin structures is very poor, whereas a model predicting muscle concentrations indicates 100% bioavailability. Regarding route, unity is likely to be surpassed with IV administration for any drug, suggesting the first dose of any drug be IV if possible. Distribution is markedly impacted by binding to plasma proteins. In general, distribution of unbound drug into tissues may approach unity to unbound drug in plasma. However, one cannot assume that only unbound drug is found in transudate or exudate as is demonstrated for cefovecin, for which binding in transudate is at least 70% and, in exudate, 90% (compared with 99% in plasma). One study attempted to measure the impact on tissue homogenate antimicrobial concentrations of negative pressure applied at the wound site.[39] Although no significant differences were reported, in fact, cefazolin tissue concentrations were always higher in the presence of negative pressure, suggesting that negative wound pressure facilitates, rather than hinders, drug distribution. One study of a cephalosporin in rats demonstrated that infection did not impact distribution (which was unity).[40] Using inflamed tissue cage models, Boothe and colleagues[41] demonstrated that accumulation of fluoroquinolones (enrofloxacin) in white blood cells increases distribution to sites of inflammation. More studies are needed to assess the impact of inflammation on antimicrobial distribution.

Biofilm

Among the factors that are likely to markedly impact therapeutic success with antimicrobials is biofilm. Bacteria exist in either a planktonic (free floating) or sessile (attached) state. It is this attached state that enables persistence of the resident population as well as the formation of biofilm.[42–45] Biofilm is defined as a biopolymer, matrix-enclosed bacterial population in which bacteria adhere either to one another

Table 2
Ratio of interstitial tissue to plasma antimicrobial concentrations

Drug	Animal	Status	Tissue	Method	Single Dose Standard	Parameter	%	Comment	Reference
Cefaclor	Rat	Normal	Lung	MicroD	Plasma (total)[a]	C_{max}	11	Ratios based on total plasma and unbound tissue. However, tissue unbound approximated 26% of plasma unbound	63
			SM			AUC	17		
						C_{max}	10		
Cefaclor	Human	Normal	SM	MicroD	Plasma (unbound)	C_{max}	38	Ratios of unbound drug ranged from 0.67 to 0.73 for immediate and modified release products	64
Cefpirome	Human	Normal	SM	MicroD	Plasma (unbound)	C_{max}	60	10% bound to plasma proteins (Muller 1997)	65
						AUC	83		
	Sepsis		SM	MicroD	Plasma (unbound)	C_{max}	38	Time to maximum concentration twice as long in septic patients	
						AUC	61		
Cefpirome	Human	Pulmonary tumors	Lung	MicroD	Plasma (total)[a]	C_{max}	42		66
						AUC	67		
Cefpirome	Human	Normal	SM	MicroD	(Total)	AUC	88	10% bound to plasma proteins	67
			SC, Adipose	MicroD		AUC	142		
Cefodizime	Human	Normal	SM	MicroD	Serum (Total)	AUC	33	74% to 89% bound to plasma proteins	67
			SC, Adipose			AUC	11		
Cefuroxime	Rabbit	Normal	Skin	MicroD	Plasma	C_{max}	10	Probe placed in superficial skin layers	68
						AUC	22		
Amoxicillin	Rabbit	Normal	Skin	MicroD	Plasma	C_{max}	6		68
						AUC	18		

Drug	Species	Condition	Tissue	Method	Sample	Parameter	Value	Notes	Ref
Amoxicillin	Rats	Normal	SM	MicroD	Plasma	NA		Predicted 80% muscle to plasma ratio with no impact of blood flow on distribution to tissue	69
Impenem	Rat	Normal	Lung SM	MicroD	Blood	C_{max} AUC C_{max} AUC	113 105 115 116		70
Imipenem	Rat	Infected with Acinetobacter	Lung Skeletal muscle	MicroD	Blood	C_{max} AUC C_{max} AUC	82 95 97 86		40
Meropenem	Dog	Normal	Subcutaneous	UltraF	Plasma (total)	AUC	138	After IV administration; 12% binding to plasma proteins	71
Cefazolin	Dog	Normal	Skin	HomoG		AUC	69	Found no statistical difference in cefazolin concentrations if wound treated with positive pressure, although numerically, concentrations were always higher, and up to 25%, in negative pressure group	39
Fosfomycin	Human	Sepsis	Skeletal muscle	MicroD	Plasma	C_{max} C_{max} AUC	69 45 68	AUC for 4 h After SQ administration;	72
Doxycycline	Dog	Normal	Subcutaneous	UltraF	Plasma (total)	AUC	17	loading dose followed by 8 h CRI half-life 4.5 h; 92% bound to plasma proteins	73
Marbofloxacin	Dog	Normal	Subcutaneous	UltraF	Plasma	AUC C_{max} AUC	213 73 111	Loading dose followed by 8 h CRI (8 h half-life); 22% bound to plasma proteins PO administration	74

(continued on next page)

Table 2
(continued)

Drug	Animal	Status	Tissue	Method	Standard	Parameter	%	Comment	Reference
Enrofloxacin	Dog	Normal	Subcutaneous	UltraF	Plasma	AUC	311	Loading dose followed by 8 h CRI (3 h half-life); 35% bound to plasma proteins	74
						C_{max}	56		
(Ciprofloxacin)[a]						C_{max}	100	(3–6 h disappearance half-life); 18.5% bound to plasma proteins	
						AUC	121		
						C_{max}	97		
						AUC	162		

Abbreviations: HomoG, homogenated tissue; MicroD, microdialysis; UltraF, ultrafiltration.
[a] Enrofloxacin also is converted to ciprofloxacin in dogs, with the active metabolite contributing up to 50% of bioactivity AUC.

or to a surface.[43] Because culture and susceptibility testing is generally implemented with bacteria in a planktonic state, data may not accurately reflect microbes existing in the sessile state in the patient.

Pathogens associated with biofilm in veterinary medicine include Acinetobacter, Actinobacillus, Klebsiella, P aeruginosa, and Staphylococcus (S aureus and S pseudintermedius). Biofilm formation has been demonstrated in canine S pseudintermedius.[5] Biofilms and their impact on veterinary medicine have been reviewed.[45]

The sophisticated organization of biofilm can present a formidable barrier to antimicrobial penetration. The outer layer of the biofilm may lose water such that it is hardened, thus providing better protection from the environment, including exposure to antimicrobials. The inner sanctum of the biofilm is largely aqueous, composed of glycocalyx or slime (eg, Staphylococcus spp). In addition to passive diffusion, aqueous pores permeate the structure, allowing movement of nutrients and metabolic debris. Using Staphylococcus spp as an example, about 85% of the biomass is a matrix in which the microbes are deeply embedded. The matrix is formed by the bacterial community, with the content varying with the bacterial species, strain, and the environment. Components include extracellular DNA (eDNA), which contributes to biofilm integrity and antimicrobial resistance.[46] Bacterial communication during biofilm formation is sophisticated, involving quorum-sensing systems that ultimately may be targets of microbial therapy.[43]

Bacterial biofilms are generally resistant to antibiotics, disinfectants, and phagocytosis. They also are largely resistant to innate and adaptive immune and inflammatory defenses.[46] For example, slime produced by Staphylococcus spp is a barrier to host defenses. Nevertheless, inflammatory cells continue to release their cytotoxic materials, contributing to host damage.[46] The steps to biofilm formation of a functional, mature biofilm include initial attachment of bacterial cells, aggregation and formation of multiple cell layers, biofilm maturation, and subsequent detachment of cells from the biofilm (platonic states) to seed formation of more biofilm.[46]

Although biofilm containing normal microflora is lost with shedding of the top most surface of cells (eg, skin or urinary bladder) or by the excretion of mucus, new cells and mucus are rapidly colonized by biofilm-forming bacteria, resulting in new (eg, persistent or recurring) infections. Microbes deep in the biofilm may contribute to chronic infection. These microbes include dormant "persister" cells that are resistant to antimicrobial therapy in their quiescent state. However, persister cells may also switch from a state of resistance to phenotypically wild-type strains for a limited period of time.[31] Because formation of persister cells appears to be stimulated by long-term, constant therapy, pulse dosing may be one approach by which their impact might be minimized.

Biofilm may facilitate and protect growth of normal or pathogenic flora on foreign surfaces and can facilitate subsequent translocation of microbes to otherwise sterile tissues. Biofilm associated with implant infections is most commonly associated with Staphylococcus spp.[46] Although not all pathogens associated with biofilm cause infection, clinical resolution of infection may not be possible until the biofilm is destroyed. Catheters (urinary or intravascular), orthopedic fixation devices, and materials used in wound management are examples of surfaces on which biofilm might develop. Stents exemplify a surface conducive to biofilm formation. Polyurethane ureteral stents in humans undergoing renal transplant were found to be positive for microbial growth 27% of the time; positive growth in all but 3% of positive infections required a sonicated fluid culture system.[47] Enterococcus spp, Staphyococcus spp, and, interestingly, Lactobacillus spp were the most common organism isolates. A higher proportion of patients with stents were bacteriuric and pyuric compared with those without, although the cause-and-effect relationship is not clear.[47]

Among the methods for achieving antimicrobial therapeutic success in the presence of biofilm is the disruption of the biofilm itself, or the use of materials that prevent biofilm formation. One approach has been the use of products that destroy the biofilm (eg, deoxyribonuclease I, which degrades eDNA or Dispersin B, which hydrolyzes N-acetylglucosamines).[46] For example, Turk and colleagues[48] demonstrated the ability of Dispersin B to penetrate the biofilm of canine methicillin-resistant S pseudintermedias. Another approach has been the use of molecules that carry antimicrobials into biofilm, thus improving delivery. However, this also increases the risk of resistance.[46] A third approach has been the use of antimicrobial-impregnated structures or application of materials that inhibit biofilm adhesion (eg, chitosan).[46] Layering of heparin as an anti-adhesive, and chitosan as an antimicrobial, is a novel approach to limiting biofilm formation on implant or other medical materials.[46] Hydroxyapatite coatings of orthopedic materials have the added advantage of not only inhibiting biofilm formation but also facilitating bone growth.

DECONTAMINATION

The risk of infection in the surgical patient is reduced, and antimicrobial de-escalation is supported by appropriate patient and surgeon antisepsis. Information addressing environmental actions to reduce SSI can be found at the Centers for Disease Control and Prevention (CDC) Healthcare Associated Infections Web site (CDC http://www.cdc.gov/HAI/ssi/ssi.html). Surgical antisepsis is defined as the application of antimicrobial chemicals to skin, mucosa, and wounds to reduce the risk of infection.[49] Surgical antisepsis most commonly involves the removal or reduction of normal flora by the topical application of antimicrobial substances to the intact skin before a surgical procedure. Distinguishing between antiseptic use on intact skin and that on mucous membranes or in wounds is important. Preparations containing alcohol or detergents (scrubs) are to be used only on intact skin. The concentration of antiseptic used in wounds is less, in general, than that of preparations applied to intact skin.

Preparation of the Skin

The purpose of a surgical hand scrub or alcohol-based hand rub is to remove transient flora and reduce resident flora for the duration of surgery in case of glove tears.[50,51] Regardless of the biocidal agent used, the technique of hand washing is important. Selection of an appropriate biocidal agent for surgical hand scrubbing should include determining what characteristics are desired, reviewing and evaluating evidence of safety and efficacy in reducing microbial counts, and considering user acceptance of the product and the costs.[50] Antiseptic treatment of the skin should not be toxic, should not cause skin reactions, and should not interfere with the normal protective function of the skin.[49] Antiseptic agents used to prepare the skin of the surgeon or patient include alcohols, chlorhexidine, iodophors, and chloroxylenols.

Alcohols, in appropriate concentrations (60%–90%), provide the most rapid and greatest reduction in microbial counts on skin.[49,50] Alcohols are not good cleansing agents, and they are not recommended in the presence of physical dirt. They should be allowed to evaporate thoroughly from the skin to be fully effective and to decrease irritation.[49] Waterless, alcohol-based hand rinse products (rubs) effectively reduce microbial counts on skin.[52] Hand rubs have been shown to be effective within application times of 90 to 180 seconds.[51] Alcohol is also used on the intact skin of the veterinary patient before surgery as a defatting agent.[53]

Chlorhexidine gluconate has both rapid and persistent antibacterial activity when used as a presurgical scrub. Its persistence is probably the best of any agent currently available for hand washing.[50] The activity of chlorhexidine is not significantly affected by blood or other organic material.[50] The incidence of skin irritation to chlorhexidine scrub seems low. Both 2% and 4% formulations in a detergent base are readily available.

Iodophors, particularly povidone-iodine, are used frequently in the presurgical preparation of surgeons and veterinary patients. The antimicrobial effects of iodophors are similar to those of iodine. Recommended levels of free iodine for antiseptics are 1 to 2 mg/L.[50] Povidone-iodine scrub has been found to be equally effective as chlorhexidine gluconate scrub in reducing the number of bacteria on canine skin for up to 1 hour after application.[54] However, bactericidal efficacy of the free iodine is bimodal, being reduced at concentrations lower and higher than recommended. Although Neihaus and colleagues[55] cited better efficacy for chlorhexidine compared with povidine-iodine as a preputial wash, the concentration of povidine-iodine was higher (25%) than recommended, potentially negating the relevance of the comparison. Iodophors are rapidly neutralized in the presence of organic materials such as blood.[50] They have a propensity toward skin irritation, and cutaneous absorption can cause thyroid dysfunction. Iodophors are available as a surgical scrub (2%) and as a solution (10% and 2%).

Chloroxylenols and bisphenols are synthetic phenol derivatives that have been used sparingly as a presurgical scrub of surgeons and veterinary patients. They are less effective than either chlorhexidine or iodophors in reducing skin flora, but chloroxylenols may have a lower incidence of skin irritation than iodophors.[50] Their activity is only minimally affected by organic matter.[50] Formulations used as a presurgical scrub include 3% chloroxylenol, 1.5% parachlorometaxylenol, and 1% to 2% triclosan.[50,56]

Preparation of Mucous Membranes

Antisepsis of mucous membranes, particularly the oral mucosa, presents particular challenges. The bacterial colonization of the oral cavity is very high, and the efficacy of oral antiseptics is affected by both dilution effects and inactivation due to salivary proteins.[57] Also, an increase in antiseptic concentration is limited by local irritation and a high absorption rate with the risk of systemic intoxication.[57] Only a few solutions are useful as oral antiseptics: povidone-iodine, chlorhexidine, and hexetidine.[57] Povidone-iodine solution has been shown to reduce inflammation and the progression of periodontal disease as well as bacteremia after dental extractions.[57]

Chlorhexidine solution is an effective agent for the prevention and treatment of oral disease.[58] Its effectiveness stems from its ability to adsorb to negatively charged surfaces in the mouth, such as the tooth and mucosa. Chlorhexidine should not, however, be used to prepare the mucous membranes of cats because of toxicity associated with erosions. Hexetidine is used as a 0.1% solution for local infections and oral hygiene. It has antimicrobial efficacy against common buccal organisms that is similar to 0.2% chlorhexidine.[59]

Wound Asepsis

When topically treating a contaminated wound with an antiseptic solution, the clinician should choose an appropriate type and concentration of antiseptic that has both antibacterial properties and minimal negative effects on wound healing. Antiseptics that appear to fulfill these criteria include chlorhexidine solution, povidone-iodine solution, and sodium hypochlorite solution (Dakin solution). Chlorhexidine diacetate solution (0.05%) has a wide spectrum of antimicrobial activity as well as minimal deleterious effects on wound healing.[60] Its sustained residual activity seems to be an advantage in wound therapy. Dilution of the stock solution with sterile water, 0.9% sodium chloride, or lactated Ringer solution does not adversely affect its antibacterial activity.[61]

Povidone-iodine solution appears to be most effective and least tissue toxic in concentrations of 0.1% to 1%.[62] Povidone-iodine concentrations greater than 0.5% are cytotoxic to the canine fibroblast in vitro.[62] Povidone-iodine should be used judiciously on large wounds because of the potential for systemic absorption of iodine.

A dilute Dakin solution (0.005% sodium hypochlorite) has been shown to be both bactericidal and not damaging to fibroblasts.[60] Dakin solution has been used as an effective irrigant for human wounds since World War I, and its use has persisted to the present. In vivo studies on the efficacy of Dakin solution in canine wounds are not available.[62]

In summary, judicious, rational antimicrobial use in the perioperative patient presents multiple challenges. The goal of therapy should not only be antimicrobial efficacy but also minimization of resistance. De-escalation of antimicrobial used involves making the appropriate decision regarding antimicrobial prophylaxis, and in the case of antimicrobial therapy, hitting hard, hitting fast, and getting out quick. Dosing regimens should be designed to kill the entire infecting inoculum, thus including selection of the antimicrobial to which the infecting isolates are most susceptible, and choosing a dose and interval that not only achieves but also ideally exceeds targeted PKPDI. Decontamination is among the most important approaches by which systemic antimicrobial use can be avoided.

REFERENCES

1. Mangram AJ, Horan TC, Pearson ML, et al. Guideline for prevention of surgical site infection, 1999. Centers for disease control and prevention (CDC) hospital infection control practices advisory committee. Am J Infect Control 1999;27:97–132.
2. Owens CD, Stoessel K. Surgical site infections: epidemiology, microbiology and prevention. J Hosp Infect 2008;70(Suppl 2):3–10.
3. Alexander JW, Solomkin JS, Edwards MJ. Updated recommendations for control of Surgical site infections. Ann Surg 2011;253:1082–93.
4. Turk R, Singh A, Weese JS. Prospective surgical site infection surveillance in dogs. Vet Surg 2014;44:2–8.
5. Singh A, Walker M, Rousseau J, et al. Characterization of the biofilm forming ability of Staphylococcus pseudintermedius from dogs. BMC Vet Res 2013;9:93.
6. Nazarali A, Singh A, Weese JS. Perioperative administration of antimicrobials during tibial plateau leveling osteotomy. Vet Surg 2014;43:966–71.
7. Schmiedt CW, Holzman G, Schwarz T, et al. Survival, complications, and analysis of risk factors after renal transplantation in cats. Vet Surg 2008;37:683–95.
8. Aly SA, Debavalya N, Suh SJ, et al. Molecular mechanisms of antimicrobial resistance in fecal Escherichia coli of healthy dogs after enrofloxacin or amoxicillin administration. Can J Microbiol 2012;58:1288–94.
9. Lawrence M, Kukanich K, Kukanich B, et al. Effect of cefovecin on the fecal flora of healthy dogs. Vet J 2013;198:259–66.
10. Bratzler DW, Dellinger EP, Olsen KM, et al. Clinical practice guidelines for antimicrobial prophylaxis in surgery. Surg Infect (Larchmt) 2013;14:73–156.
11. Boothe DM. Principles of Antimicrobial Therapy. In: Boothe DM, editor. Small Animal Clinical Pharmacology and Therapeutics. 2nd edition. Philadelphia: Elsevier; 2012. p. 128–78.

12. Githaiga A, Ndirangu M, Paterson DL. Infections in the immunocompromised patient. In: Fink MP, Abraham E, Vincent E, et al, editors. Textbook of critical care. 5th edition. Philadelphia: Saunders; 2005.

13. Eugster S, Schawalder P, Gaschen F, et al. A prospective study of postoperative surgical site infections in dogs and cats. Vet Surg 2004;33:542–50.

14. Thungrat KT, Carpenter M, Boothe DM. Antimicrobial susceptibility patterns of clinical Escherichia coli isolates from dogs and cats in the United States: January 2008 through January 2013. Vet Microbiol 2014.

15. Weese JS, van Duijkeren E. Methicillin-resistant Staphylococcus aureus and Staphylococcus pseudintermedius in veterinary medicine. Vet Microbiol 2010; 140:418–29.

16. Hawn MT, Richman JS, Vick CC, et al. Timing of surgical antibiotic prophylaxis and the risk of surgical site infection. JAMA Surg 2013;148:649–57.

17. Stegemann MR, Sherington J, Blanchflower S. Pharmacokinetics and pharmacodynamics of cefovecin in dogs. J Vet Pharmacol Ther 2006;29:501–11.

18. Daude-Lagrave A, Carozzo C, Fayolle P, et al. Infection rates in surgical procedures: a comparison of cefalexin vs. a placebo. Vet Comp Orthop Traumatol 2001;14(3):146–50.

19. Hettlich BF, Boothe HW, Simpson RB, et al. Effect of tympanic cavity evacuation and flushing on microbial isolates during total ear canal ablation with lateral bulla osteotomy in dogs. J Am Vet Med Assoc 2005;227:748–55.

20. McHugh SM, Collins CJ, Corrigan MA, et al. The role of topical antibiotics used as prophylaxis in surgical site infection prevention. J Antimicrob Chemother 2011; 66:693–701.

21. Huiras P, Logan JK, Papadopoulos S, et al. Local antimicrobial administration for prophylaxis of surgical site infections. Pharmacotherapy 2001;32:1006–19.

22. Atilla A, Boothe HW, Tollett M, et al. In vitro elution of amikacin and vancomycin from impregnated plaster of Paris beads. Vet Surg 2010;39:715–21.

23. Phillips H, Boothe DM, Shofer F, et al. In vitro elution studies of amikacin and cefazolin from polymethylmethacrylate. Vet Surg 2007;36:272–8.

24. Ham K, Griff D, Seddighi M, et al. Clinical application of tobramycin-impregnated calcium sulfate beads in six dogs (2002-2004). J Am Anim Hosp Assoc 2008;44: 320–6.

25. Sayegh AI, Moore RM. Polymethylmethacrylate beads for treating orthopedic infections. Compend Contin Educ Pract Vet 2003;25:788–95.

26. Neut D, van de Belt H, Stokroos I, et al. Biomaterial-associated infection of gentamicin-loaded PMMA beads in orthopaedic revision surgery. J Antimicrob Chemother 2001;47:885–91.

27. Owen MR, Moores AP, Cox RJ. Management of MRSA septic arthritis in a dog using a gentamicin-impregnated collagen sponge. J Small Anim Pract 2004;45: 609–12.

28. Mealey KL, Boothe DM. Nephrotoxicosis associated with topical administration of gentamicin in a cat. J Am Vet Med Assoc 1994;204:1919–21.

29. Rossolini GM, Arena F, Pecile P, et al. Update on the antibiotic resistance crisis. Curr Opin Pharmacol 2014;18C:56–60.

30. Mouton JW, Ambrose PG, Canton R, et al. Conserving antibiotics for the future: new ways to use old and new drugs from a pharmacokinetic and pharmacodynamic perspective. Drug Resist Updat 2011;14:107–17.

31. Martinez MN, Papich MG, Drusano GL. Dosing regimen matters: the importance of early intervention and rapid attainment of the pharmacokinetic/pharmacodynamics target. Antimicrob Agents Chemother 2012;56:2795–805.

32. Liu X, Boothe DM, Jin Y, et al. In vitro potency and efficacy favor later generation fluoroquinolones for treatment of canine and feline Escherichia coli uropathogens in the United States. World J Microbiol Biotechnol 2013;29:347–54.

33. Ryan DM. Pharmacokinetics of antibiotics in natural and experimental superficial compartments in animals and humans. J Antimicrob Chemother 1993;31(Suppl D):1–16.

34. Barza M. Tissue directed antibiotic therapy: antibiotic dynamics in cells and tissues. Clin Infect Dis 1994;19:910–5.

35. Müller M, dela Peña A, Derendorf H. Issues in pharmacokinetics and pharmacodynamics of anti-infective agents: distribution in tissue. Antimicrob Agents Chemother 2004;48:1441–53.

36. Bamberger DM, Foxworth JW, Bridewell DL, et al. Extravascular antimicrobial distribution and the respective blood and urine concentrations in humans. In: Lorian V, editor. Antibiotics in laboratory medicine. Baltimore (MD): Williams & Wilkins; 2005. p. 719–848.

37. Boothe DM, Boeckh A, Boothe HW, et al. Tissue concentrations of enrofloxacin and ciprofloxacin in anesthetized dogs following single intravenous administration. Vet Ther 2001;2:120–8.

38. Brunner M, Derendorf H, Müller M. Microdialysis for in vivo pharmacokinetic/pharmacodynamic characterization of anti-infective drugs. Curr Opin Pharmacol 2005;5:495–9.

39. Coutin JV, Lanz OI, Magnin-Bissel GC, et al. Cefazolin concentration in surgically created wounds treated with negative pressure wound therapy compared to surgically created wounds treated with nonadherent wound dressings. Vet Surg 2015;44:9–16.

40. Dahyot C, Marchand S, Pessini GL, et al. Microdialysis study of imipenem distribution in skeletal muscle and lung extracellular fluids of Acinetobacter baumannii-infected rats. Antimicrob Agents Chemother 2006;50:2265–7.

41. Boothe DM, Boeckh A, Boothe HW. Evaluation of the distribution of enrofloxacin by circulating leukocytes to sites of inflammation in dogs. Am J Vet Res 2009;70: 16–22.

42. Clutterbuck AL, Woods EJ, Knottenbelt DC, et al. Biofilms and their relevance to veterinary medicine. Vet Microbiol 2007;121:1–17.

43. Hentzer M, Eberl L, Nielsen J, et al. Quorum sensing: a novel target for the treatment of biofilm infections. BioDrugs 2003;17:241–50.

44. Marsh PD. Dental plaque: biological significance of a biofilm and community lifestyle. J Clin Periodontol 2005;32(Suppl 6):7–15.

45. Percival SL, Knottenbelt DC, Cochrane CA, editors. Biofilms and veterinary medicine. Heidelberg (Germany); Dordrecht (Netherlands); New York: Springer; 2011.

46. Arciola CR, Campoccia D, Speziale P, et al. Biofilm formation in Staphylococcus implant infections. A review of molecular mechanisms and implications for biofilm-resistant materials. Biomaterials 2012;33:5967–82.

47. Bonkat G, Rieken M, Siegel FP, et al. Microbial ureteral stent colonization in renal transplant recipients: frequency and influence on the short-time functional outcome. Transpl Infect Dis 2012;14:57–63.

48. Turk R, Singh A, Rousseau J, et al. In vitro evaluation of DispersinB on methicillin-resistant Staphylococcus pseudintermedius biofilm. Vet Microbiol 2013;166(3–4): 576–9.

49. Crabtree TD, Pelletier SJ, Pruett TL. Surgical antisepsis. In: Block SS, editor. Disinfection, sterilization, and preservation. 5th edition. Philadelphia: Lippincott Williams & Wilkins; 2001. p. 919.

50. Larson EL. APIC guideline for handwashing and hand antisepsis in health care settings. Am J Infect Control 1995;23:251–69.
51. Suchomel M, Gnant G, Weinlich M, et al. Surgical hand disinfection using alcohol: the effects of alcohol type, mode and duration of application. J Hosp Infect 2009; 71:228–33.
52. Larson EL, Aiello AE, Heilman JM, et al. Comparison of different regimens for surgical hand preparation. AORN J 2001;73:412–20.
53. Shmon C. Assessment and preparation of the surgical patient and the operating team. In: Slatter D, editor. Textbook of small animal surgery. 3rd edition. Philadelphia: Saunders; 2003. p. 162.
54. Osuna DJ, DeYoung DJ, Walker RL. Comparison of three skin preparation techniques in the dog. Part I: Experimental trial. Vet Surg 1990;19:14–9.
55. Neihaus SA, Hathcock TL, Boothe DM, et al. Presurgical antiseptic efficacy of chlorhexidine diacetate and providone-iodine in the canine preputial cavity. J Am Anim Hosp Assoc 2011;47:406–12.
56. Kampf G, Kramer A. Epidemiologic background of hand hygiene and evaluation of the most important agents for scrubs and rubs. Clin Microbiol Rev 2004;17: 863–93.
57. Rahn R. Review presentation on povidone-iodine antisepsis in the oral cavity. Postgrad Med J 1993;69:S4–9.
58. Denton GW. Chlorhexidine. In: Block SS, editor. Disinfection, sterilization, and preservation. 5th edition. Philadelphia: Lippincott Williams & Wilkins; 2001. p. 321.
59. Ashley KC. The antimicrobial properties of two commonly used antiseptic mouthwashes—corsodyl and oraldene. J Appl Bacteriol 1984;56:221–5.
60. Swaim SF, Lee AH. Topical wound medications: a review. J Am Vet Med Assoc 1987;190:1588–93.
61. Lozier S, Pope E, Berg J. Effects of four preparations of 0.05% chlorhexidine diacetate on wound healing in dogs. Vet Surg 1992;21:107–12.
62. Lemarié RJ, Hosgood G. Antiseptics and disinfectants in small animal practice. Compend Contin Educ Pract Vet 1995;17:1339–51.
63. de La Peña A, Dalla Costa T, Talton JD, et al. Penetration of cefaclor into the interstitial space fluid of skeletal muscle and lung tissue in rats. Pharm Res 2001;18: 1310–4.
64. de La Peña A, Brunner M, Eichler HG, et al. Comparative target site pharmacokinetics of immediate- and modified-release formulations of cefaclor in humans. J Clin Pharmacol 2002;42:403–11.
65. Joukhadar C, Klein N, Mayer BX, et al. Plasma and tissue pharmacokinetics of cefpirome in patients with sepsis. Crit Care Med 2002;7:1478–82.
66. Herkner H, Müller MR, Kreischitz N, et al. Closed-chest microdialysis to measure antibiotic penetration into human lung tissue. Am J Respir Crit Care Med 2002; 165:273–6.
67. Müller M, Rohde B, Kovar A, et al. Relationship between serum and free interstitial concentrations of cefodizime and cefpirome in muscle and subcutaneous adipose tissue of healthy volunteers measured by microdialysis. J Clin Pharmacol 1997;37:1108–13.
68. Shukla C, Patel V, Juluru R, et al. Quantification and prediction of skin pharmacokinetics of amoxicillin and cefuroxime. Biopharm Drug Dispos 2009;30:281–93.
69. Marchand S, Chenel M, Lamarche I, et al. Pharmacokinetic modeling of free amoxicillin concentrations in rat muscle extracellular fluids determined by microdialysis. Antimicrob Agents Chemother 2005;49:3702–6.

70. Marchand S, Dahyot C, Lamarche I, et al. Microdialysis study of imipenem distribution in skeletal muscle and lung extracellular fluids of noninfected rats. Antimicrob Agents Chemother 2005;49:2356–61.
71. Bidgood T, Papich MG. Plasma pharmacokinetics and tissue fluid concentrations of meropenem after intravenous and subcutaneous administration in dogs. Am J Vet Res 2002;63:1622–8.
72. Matzi V, Lindenmann J, Porubsky C, et al. Extracellular concentrations of fosfomycin in lung tissue of septic patients. J Antimicrob Chemother 2010;65:995–8.
73. Bidgood TL, Papich MG. Comparison of plasma and interstitial fluid concentrations of doxycycline and meropenem following constant rate intravenous infusion in dogs. Am J Vet Res 2003;64:1040–6.
74. Bidgood TL, Papich MG. Plasma and interstitial fluid pharmacokinetics of enrofloxacin, its metabolite ciprofloxacin, and marbofloxacin after oral administration and a constant rate intravenous infusion in dogs. J Vet Pharmacol Ther 2005;28:329–41.

Index

Note: Page numbers of article titles are in **boldface** type.

Moving?

Make sure your subscription moves with you!

To notify us of your new address, find your **Clinics Account Number** (located on your mailing label above your name), and contact customer service at:

Email: journalscustomerservice-usa@elsevier.com

800-654-2452 (subscribers in the U.S. & Canada)
314-447-8871 (subscribers outside of the U.S. & Canada)

Fax number: 314-447-8029

Elsevier Health Sciences Division
Subscription Customer Service
3251 Riverport Lane
Maryland Heights, MO 63043

*To ensure uninterrupted delivery of your subscription, please notify us at least 4 weeks in advance of move.

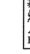
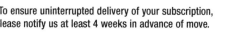